Supervision of Midwives

Edited by
Mavis Kirkham

Books for Midwives Press
An imprint of Hochland & Hochland Ltd

Published by Books for Midwives Press, 174a Ashley Road, Hale, Cheshire, WA15 9SF, England.

ISBN 1-898507-14-7

British Library Cataloguing in Publication Data
A catalogue record for this book is available from the British Library

Printed in Great Britain by Redwood Books, Trowbridge, Wiltshire

Contents

Audit

Research: Midwives' Views of Supervision

Using the Experience of Other Professions

Introduction

Mavis Kirkham RGN, RM, BA, MA, PhD, Cert Ed (Adult), FP Nursing Cert
is currently Professor of Midwifery at the University of Sheffield. She has 20 years of experience of clinical midwifery and research and five years of midwifery education.

This book about the supervision of midwives has much in common with its subject: whilst it is concerned with one issue, its contents are highly diverse. This is not an academic tome though it contains a number of chapters of research findings. I would like to compare it, and supervision, with a rich patchwork quilt. Its chapters differ in size, texture and content. Some chapter authors are eminent professional figures and a number are writing for publication for the first time. Some report on research or audit and some seek to bring local innovations into the arena of professional debate. Some chapters are cheering, some are sad. There are inevitably very different viewpoints. There are dissonances and conflicting views between chapters as there are differences in views between supervisors and between midwives and contradictions inherent in the very role of supervisor of midwives.

Why this book now?

Midwifery is in a time of great change. There are real opportunities and many dilemmas following from 'Changing Childbirth' (Department of Health, 1993) and recent changes in the National Health Service. In order to seize these opportunities with due regard for the dilemmas there is a great need to facilitate planned change for the benefit of childbearing women and to which midwives feel a real commitment. To achieve such tasks we must work with appropriately well honed tools. One of the tools available is clearly the statutory supervision of midwives. Yet that tool dates from a very different era and was designed for very different work. It therefore seemed right to bring together the knowledge, views and experiences of some of those supervising midwives, being supervised as midwives, thinking about, researching and auditing the supervision of midwives within this book.

There have been articles on supervision, more recently there have been dissertations and conference proceedings. This is the first edited book on this subject. We see this as the start of a published debate.

This book is concerned primarily with the supervision of midwives in England, except for Jane Winship's Chapter 3 which takes a UK perspective. We hope the book will stimulate discussion on the subject throughout the United Kingdom and beyond.

Background

The supervision of midwives was designed to control the practice of midwives, most of whom worked independently and were often isolated in an era when this control was felt to be highly important by the medical profession, which controlled midwifery and by the 'ladies' who sought to reform midwifery practice (Brooke Heagerty, Chapter 1). Now there are many mechanisms to control midwifery, most midwives are employees, 'communication systems are rapid and very powerful' (Jenkins, 1995) and supervision is seen in a very different light by the United Kingdom Central Council for Nursing, Midwifery and Health Visiting (UKCC), as enabling rather than controlling midwifery practice (see Chapter 3). Yet the structures have changed very little and we are affected by our history. The many changes of recent years have contained threats as well as opportunities for midwives. In times of threat and weariness with change, we reasonably hang on to what we have and statutory supervision is something unique to midwifery. Nevertheless we need to be sure that what we have is fit for its purpose otherwise there is a danger that we ride the dinosaur we know and love in a race where others have more responsive and streamlined steeds.

Ironically, whilst statutory supervision is unique to midwifery and has a long history, midwives are remarkably ignorant about the nature and purpose of supervision as is demonstrated in a number of chapters in this book. Yet an understanding of the supervisory relationship is fundamental if we are to make the most of that relationship.

The supervisory relationship

The supervision of midwives exists both to prevent bad practice and to promote good practice. Over the years the emphasis has moved from the former to the latter aspects of the role but both remain. Different skills are required for these two functions and the vigilance which was traditionally applied to root out bad practice is very different from the support skills needed to foster the confidence in the face of uncertainty which is needed for innovation. There is inherently a tension between the 'policeman and friend' aspects of supervisor's role (ARM, 1995), indeed some see them as separate roles or as aspects of supervision which could be practised with different supervisees. Rosemary Johnson (Chapter 7) stresses that where there are investigations of alleged poor practice 'it is important that the midwife has access to a named supervisor who is independent of the investigation and can provide support'.

The structures which were set up to control midwifery at the beginning of this century must now be seen as unjust (Brooke Heagerty, Chapter 1). Considerable changes have been made to correct this; for instance concerning disciplinary proceedings against midwives, though some would say that further reforms are needed. Similarly with supervision considerable changes have been made (see Chapters 3 and 4), though changes may not always equate with progress (see Chapter 2). The attention now being given to the preparation of supervisors (see Chapter 4) and the procedures for selection and deselection (Chapter 3) give clear evidence of a will to improve supervision. It could, however, be argued that this process is still in its early stages and the real heart of the matter is concerned with what happens within the supervisory relationship and the exercise of power within that relationship. Until this is addressed it could be argued that there is 'no appeal' (Cathy Shennan, Chapter 12) against supervisory decisions which involve only the supervisor and supervisee. In the terms used by Ruth Deery and Debi Corby (Chapter 14) to describe clinical supervision this means that there is no 'safety' in the relationship.

The silent nature of good supervision

There are considerable problems in examining the supervision of midwives because of the 'silent' (Page, 1995) nature of good supervision: if midwives are empowered by supervision then the visible achievements are by the supervisee, not the supervisor. In this there is a direct parallel with the nature of good midwifery practice which helps childbearing women towards achievements which are theirs and not their midwife's.

Lack of awareness of the nature of facilitation or empowerment has led to much criticism of published work on supervision as being negative or not telling the good stories of supervision. The good stories, by definition, would be stories of midwifery, not of supervision.

Parallel processes

Parallel processes can be seen in the relationship between supervisor and supervisee and that between supervisee and client, as identified by Eckstein and Wallenstein (1958) or as conveyed in the truism 'as midwives are cared for so do they care for women'.

The nature of the relationship between the midwife and her client has changed greatly since 1902. Earlier this century the very detailed Midwives Rules and general social expectations meant that midwives, to a considerable extent, controlled the childbearing experiences of their clients. Onto this was transposed a medical model of childbearing where control of process and therefore of experience was central (Arney, 1982), alongside the organizational controls of institutionalized childbearing. Recently there have been political changes in society which are now becoming manifest in relationships between clients and professional caregivers. 'Changing Childbirth' (Department of Health, 1993) stresses choice and control for childbearing women. The question therefore arises as to how far existing models of the supervision of midwives enable midwives to experience and find role models for the empowering, equal relationships which they are now required to foster with their clients. If midwives are to be able to empower women, they themselves must be empowered (Cathy Warwick, Chapter 8). The chapters in the *Examples of Good Practice* section of this book (Chapters 6-8) address this issue in varying ways.

It is significant that it is Helen Lewison, in examining supervision as a public service (Chapter 5), who uses the Midwifery Relationships section of the International Code of Ethics for Midwives (ICM, 1993) to examine this issue. She highlights key areas of skill where supervisors can act as role models: the utilization of peer support and conflict resolution are key examples.

In terms of the present aims of supervision as enabling midwives to facilitate choice and control for their clients, parallel processes can be seen which have negative results. Elizabeth Williams describes an informal supervisory network which maintains the organizational hierarchy. It could be that it was the hierarchical hospital structures within which they worked which led to some midwives in that study shifting responsibility for their practice onto their supervisor. It is ironic that when midwifery nationally aims to facilitate choice and control for clients, Cathy Shennan found midwives who saw their supervisors as needing to have their control of midwives decision-making acknowledged. This caused dependence in those who needed role models to themselves facilitate autonomy. It is likely that those supervisors needed this because their own experience was of being controlled and defence reactions had been developed as a result of such experience.

Trust and support are clearly key issues in the supervision of midwives and are raised in most chapters of this book. Meg Taylor sees the trust of colleagues as essential if midwives are to develop 'a repertoire of flexible responses' which form the basis of autonomous clinical judgement. Yet midwifery does not have a culture where we can express our need for trust and support. With regard to psychological and physical resources Meg Taylor states:

> '...it is a basic tenet of counselling that I cannot be expected to give to my client if I don't have enough resources for myself. Counsellors are expected to make sure they have enough resources to function. This requires a kind of self-centredness which is not egotism but which ultimately serves the interests of the client'.

How can we facilitate clients in voicing their needs whilst suppressing our own needs as midwives? This is particularly evident around coping with stress which, with skilled support and facilitation, can be used to increase our understanding of ourselves and our clients. If we lack such skilled help stress leads us to create the rigid defence mechanism from which we seek to free ourselves.

Supervisors also have needs, indeed their role puts heavy pressures upon them. The question of who supports the supervisors is raised in many chapters of this book but satisfactory answer are few. It is perhaps not surprising that some of the midwives Cathy Shennan studied spoke of supervisors 'down-loading their problems onto midwives'. Without starting with good support for supervisors it seems unreasonable to ask them to role model skills in facilitation and support which they themselves do not experience.

Meg Taylor and Jill Demilew see the aim of good supervision being to 'midwife the midwife' in terms of support and parallel processes. Clearly it is equally important to 'midwife' and 'supervise' the supervisor. If this does not happen the rigidities of the past will continue to be reproduced.

Differing philosophies of midwifery

Several chapters in this book demonstrate in very different settings that a supervisor is perceived as good where she shares a similar philosophy of practice with those she supervises. Conversely, supervision is poor where there are very different professional philosophies and the supervisor's efforts to work according to her philosophy, backed by the power of her position as supervisor, is perceived as controlling. In such a situation it is highly unlikely that the supervisor can facilitate improvements in practice because of the differing values upon which practice is built. It is noteworthy that Elizabeth Williams (Chapter 11) found this in her study of NHS midwives as did Jill Demilew (Chapter 13) in her study of independent midwives. It may well be that the much publicised problems which independent midwives have experienced with supervision are due to this difference in philosophy between them and their supervisors, all of whom are employed by the NHS and most of whom are senior managers, rather than to their being independent midwives.

Elizabeth Williams concludes that those whose views are on the periphery or who 'display levels of attitudinal autonomy which are outside the socially accepted norm' may find themselves in conflict with their supervisors. Whilst this is not surprising, it is worrying, for surely those at the forefront of change are in just this position as were independent midwives before 'Changing Childbirth' (Department of Health, 1993) set continuity of care as a standard to which we are all required to aspire. Questions then arise as to the relationship between supervision and innovation and the extent to which supervision could be an inherently conservative element in a changing world of clinical practice.

It is useful here to look at the findings of Jill Demilew and Elizabeth Williams alongside the innovations described by Kate Caldwell and Cathy Warwick. The latter are clearly building mechanisms of supervision and staff support which facilitate fundamental changes in the locus of power and control between supervisor and supervisee and between midwife and mother. Supervision built on such a philosophy is likely to be supportive to innovations within the basic philosophy of choice and control for childbearing women. This fits the analysis of Jill Demilew and Elizabeth Williams that the important issue in successful supervision is a shared philosophy of practice between supervisor and supervisee.

Whilst it is easy to see problems where midwives have embraced the philosophy of facilitating choice and control for women and their supervisors take the controlling stance of an earlier philosophy of midwifery practice, this problem can also be seen in reverse. Supervision can be used to facilitate change in the philosophy of practice as is demonstrated in Chapters 6-8.

Supervision and management

Since supervision moved into hospital structures (see Chapter 2) supervisors have usually also been midwifery managers. This dual role creates tensions between the management aim of organizing a workforce economically on behalf of an employer and the supervisory aims of protecting the public and enabling midwives to develop their practice (the tensions between these latter two aims have been noted above). McDowell (1993) found that some supervisors have difficulty in differentiating between the managerial and supervisory aspects of their work. That difficulty is also evident in some chapters of this book. It is therefore not surprising that some midwives were confused as to the roles of manager and supervisor. Misunderstandings around the vexed issue of 'suspension' are a good example of this confusion (see Chapter 12).

Efforts have been made in some settings to separate the roles of supervisor and manager. Jean Duerden (Chapter 10) found, in some of the units she audited, that supervisors did not supervise midwives whom they managed. She calls this 'cross supervision'.

Some units now have supervisors who hold E or F grade posts which are clinical and not managerial. Glynnis Mayes and Meryl Thomas (Chapter 4) see this as a positive move in 'demonstrating that supervision is quite separate from management and giving more credibility to practitioners'. Yet a management role, whilst it may provide conflicting allegiances with the supervisor's role, also gives the supervisor the opportunity to initiate change or influence others in directions which she as a supervisor feels are important. What Glennis Mayes and Meryl Thomas describe as 'this balance between the professional practice issues central to the supervisory role and the employment, cost effective and expediency focus of the management role that successful supervisors have been able to achieve' is clearly of political importance for midwifery as is the need to influence policy at both trust and purchaser level. Clearly E and F grade supervisors will have little opportunity to have influence in these areas of political importance for midwifery. Conversely it is doubtful that an E grade midwife with a short term or bank contract will feel truly free to discuss with her supervisor the weaker points she has identified in her practice when that supervisor is also the manager she seeks to impress to gain a permanent contract. It is of interest that Jean Duerden, in her recommendations arising from her audit of supervision, states that 'the minimum grade for a supervisor should be grade G'.

So as well as the policeman and friend tensions within the role of supervisor, there appears to be another role of politician or leader which creates further intra-role tensions. The supervisor has to be a leader in the sense of being a valued role model to those she supervises. Yet if she is in a position to hold sufficient power to really have a positive influence on behalf of midwifery in wider forums this may well reduce her effectiveness in the friend and counsellor aspect of her role because of her identification with the employer in the minds of midwives.

Supervision can also develop issues raised in a management context. Kate Caldwell describes supervision as a context in which to discuss the way forward from professional objectives raised in individual performance review. The resources needed for change, especially for education, are of course controlled by management. But it may well expand horizons to discuss issues identified in a management context in the wider context of supervision before addressing issues of funding.

Whilst the tensions between supervision and management are real, there are now considerably fewer midwifery managers as a result of both cuts, over which midwives had little control, and deliberate choice to create structures which are less hierarchical with more autonomy for clinicians. This flattening management structure has implications for supervision in several of its aspects. Cathy Warwick sees supervision as more important now that midwives are less closely managed. It is certainly logical that as the management hierarchy flattens such a facilitating relationship should come to the fore and could even provide a safe setting in which to dissolve some defence mechanisms. Glynnis Mayes and Meryl Thomas look at flattening managerial structures in the context of the need for professional leadership 'at clinical, Trust Board and purchasing authority level'. It is worth considering how far supervisors can become professional leaders without creating a new hierarchy.

It is ironic that many of the new facilitative concepts being applied in supervision are also being used in modern management. This is very much the case with empowerment (Judge, 1996) which can be a two edged weapon for employees. Thus management, which many seek to separate from supervision, is developing in the same direction as supervision. It is interesting to note that Cathy Warwick in another context (Warwick, 1996) addressing midwifery management highlights many of the issues raised here in considering supervision:

> 'It is ludicrous to expect midwives to be responsible and autonomous in practice and yet as employees to treat them as children... It is tempting to fall back in the climate of risk management on tight control but this will not result in service change' (Warwick, 1996, p.229).

Strategies for empowerment

It is cheering to see such similar statements in this book as to how good supervision can be achieved. In the discussions of innovations in the practice of supervision openness, honesty and trust are seen as the key to enabling 'midwives to grow and develop' (Cathy Warwick). These authors are aware of the operation of parallel processes at a very practical level. Kate Caldwell aims 'to encourage a feeling of well-being and a sense of being valued' amongst midwives who will then be equipped to build similar valuing relationships with their clients. The 'Care for the Carers' programme in Exeter, aims to equip individuals to identify and deal with stress and provides a range of opportunities for professional and personal support.

Cathy Warwick states that 'Normally... high standards will emerge more effectively if midwives are treated themselves as they are expected to treat women'. She looks at supervision in the context of practice change at King's and focuses on the key areas where support is required and can be given proactively through planned 'mechanisms of support'. The change in the locus of power inherent in team midwifery is fostered: 'decisions about change always come from the midwives themselves and the role of the supervisor is to facilitate discussion and introduce ideas, not to impose solutions'. Rosemary Johnson described how supervision in Southmead was tailored to the needs of midwives and the service they now provide. The issue of support is examined in detail and she gives examples of how midwives were involved in policy formulation and facilitated in exercising choice. Inevitably choice leads to dilemmas and the issue of midwives who do not accept the invitation to a supervisory interview is honestly aired. This opens up wider areas of trust concerning supervision. Elizabeth Williams found that few of the midwives she studied wished to choose their supervisors, though those studied by Jean Duerden did. Meg Taylor (Chapter 15) takes up this issue of lack of trust amongst midwives and concludes:

> '... this lack of trust reflects the punitive and persecutory nature of the midwifery hierarchy and its ethos.
>
> When aggression is projected outwards onto others, there is an unconscious fear that it will return, aimed at oneself.
>
> I also feel that this mistrust is an expression of the contempt which midwives have for themselves and for others and which is an internalization of their inferior position with regard to obstetrics.'

She sees supervision in counselling as emotionally difficult but 'ultimately strengthening' and asks:

> 'Could an analogous system midwife midwives through the transition from a hierarchy which encourages delegation upwards to a more egalitarian network structure which will both foster and reflect clinical autonomy?'

Midwives do not practise alone and supervisors can empower midwives in their relationships with other professions. Cathy Warwick discussed techniques by which this can be achieved within the overall philosophy of present practice at King's and there are examples of supervisors acting as advocates for midwives with other professions throughout the book.

Clinical supervision

In the view of the UKCC, clinical supervision 'brings practitioners and skilled supervisors together to reflect on practice'. The aim is 'to identify solutions to problems, improve practice and increase understanding of professional issues'. It is not 'a managerial control system' and is not 'hierarchical in nature' (UKCC, 1996). Ruth Deery and Debi Corby's definition (Chapter 14) links with Rogers' definition of counselling and both stress trust, safety and development. Tensions between this situation and the supervisor who is appointed to be 'over' the midwife rather than 'with' her are highlighted in Chapter 14, alongside the external pressures which restrict the supervisor's ability to provide the safe relationship required in clinical supervision. Ruth Deery and Debi Corby therefore conclude that 'supervisors of midwives are not in the best position to act as clinical supervisors as it places unfair and unforeseen demands upon them'. Nevertheless, in the view of the UKCC (1996), 'clinical supervision is an integral part of the role of the supervisor of midwives'.

It is ironic that the most obvious difference between the supervision of midwives and clinical supervision concerns the 'policing' role in midwifery supervision. Yet the responsibilities of the supervisor when bad practice is suspected are anticipated and clearly negotiated prior to clinical supervision in other professions (Butterworth and Faugier, 1992).

It is significant that at Exeter and at King's both counselling and clinical supervision are available to midwives as part of their support services in addition to statutory supervision.

Standards and audit

There has been, and still is, much confusion about supervision in the minds of midwives and supervisors. In seeking to improve midwifery services and to change supervision so that it can more effectively underpin and facilitate those changes, a clear picture of supervision is needed. Clear procedures and guidelines for all aspects of supervision can promote understanding without reducing flexibility. Rosemary Johnson stresses the need for clearly laid out procedures around the investigation of alleged poor practice.

Once there are clear guidelines and procedures it is essential that they are audited. Ann Skipworth (Chapter 10) describes the formulation and introduction of ten standards for supervisors in the West Midlands and the subsequent audit of those standards. By choosing a process by which supervisors audited supervisors from another district it is clear that the actual process of audit was a learning experience for all those involved. Though problems are honestly reported and philosophies of control were seen in some places, the potential for supervisors to learn through this process 'in a non-threatening environment' is clearly demonstrated. This process appears to have helped some supervisors to develop a proactive approach to supervision. Here is another imaginative and fruitful way of improving the practice of supervision. It was difficult to decide whether Chapter 10 fitted best under the heading of 'Audit' or 'Examples of good practice'; another example of the multifaceted nature of supervision.

Jean Duerden (Chapter 10) conducted an audit of supervision throughout the area of the North West Regional Health Authority. She provides a clear picture of how supervision is organized over a large geographical area and goes on to state honestly that 'the quality of the supervisory review also needs assessing'. The role of supervisor as supporter was identified as the most important aspect of supervision to all the groups involved in this audit. The difficulties of the role in the face of the 137 different areas of support required by midwives are also explored. It is significant that the majority of the midwives there wanted to be able to choose their supervisor and the practical issues around this are explored.

Supervision in the wider context

In its concern with the practice of midwives the supervision of midwives is also involved with other groups. The welfare of the childbearing family is at the heart of the supervisor's concerns. In this context it is interesting to note the differing attitudes within this book to the relationship between supervision and the maternity service user. Helen Lewison

(Chapter 5), taking the user's viewpoint, is clear that supervision should be in the background to the primary relationship between the midwife and the childbearing woman and that any action by the supervisor to change that risks disempowering the primary relationship. The midwife authors of other chapter have very different views. Rosemary Johnson (Chapter 7) argues very clearly that where there are problems an interview between the mother, her partner, her midwife and the supervisor should be offered to enable 'the supervisor to be an informed advocate for the mother and baby' in circumstances where the mother is at risk of 'feeling totally disempowered', as well as supporting the midwife.

There is also the question of the supervision of midwives and the wider social context of women's lives. In Helen Lewison's view 'It is for supervisors to take the lead in campaigning for better midwifery provision for all women'. This ties in with the picture of supervision in Nottingham 1948-72 given by Julia Allison and myself. It is another of the ironies of the history of supervision that at the time when the supervision of midwives moved into the control of midwives, it also moved out the wider public health context of women's lives.

Inter-professional relationships are of great importance in midwifery and the nature of these relationships needs to change as the nature of midwifery practice changes. Cathy Warwick describes how this has been achieved at King's. She states that, 'It is through reflection on cases that most is learned about inter-professional working'. The monthly meeting with supervisors there allows midwives to reflect on midwifery practice, informs the supervisor of the state of relationships with other professions and equips her to act as an advocate for her midwives. The supervisors role with regard to other professions is raised in a number of chapters concerning the present and Julia Allison and myself give a good example from the past.

Dilemmas: Community of roles

What is expected of the supervisor of midwives is not that she adopt one clear role. There is a whole community of roles (Mair, 1977) in the concept of supervision. Some of the roles date from different historical eras and are rooted in different philosophies of practice. There are differing degrees of compatibility between these roles. Some appear to be inherently in conflict and some support each other. An examination of these different roles and their relationship with each other would prove immensely fruitful for midwifery and for the practice of individual supervisors. Once the different roles are examined it is possible to examine how they can relate better to each other. It is also possible to question how far all supervisors can be active in all of these roles. It could be that too much is contained within supervision and that it is not possible for supervision to achieve all that has been added to its aims over the years. For the present, however, it is important to make the most of what we have. The concept of a community of supervisory roles may prove useful in that it implies change and mutual adaptation within the supervisory roles as well as with supervisees and others. The complex relationships and the potential conflicts within supervision must be consciously addressed and developed to best advantage by each supervisor in her own situation. This is a continuous process of development and adaptation.

The relationship between supervision and midwifery education is crucial here. The midwifery teacher and supervisor who was to address this issue in the book withdrew from the project when it was too late to replace her. This inevitably leaves a gap which must be addressed in the future.

The English National Board for Nursing, Midwifery and Health Visiting has just commissioned a piece of research, partly funded by the UKCC, to examine the supervision of midwives and to evaluate its impact on professional practice and the quality of midwifery care in England. Those of us involved in this research see it as a key opportunity to take forward the analysis of supervision and thereby its development.

Meanwhile we seek to develop midwifery care and supervision. It is appropriate that as we develop new ways of providing midwifery care, we also develop more appropriate ways of 'midwifing the midwife'.

References

Association of Radical Midwives (1995). *Super-Vision: Consensus Conference Proceedings.* Hale: Books for Midwives Press.

Arney, W.R. (1982). *Power and the Profession of Obstetrics.* Chicago: University of Chicago Press.

Butterworth, T., Faugier, J. (1992). *Clinical Supervision.* London: Chapman and Hall.

Department of Health (1993). *Changing Childbirth.* London: HMSO.

Duerden, J. (1995) *Audit of Supervision of Midwives in the North West Regional Health Authority.* Salford Royal Hospitals NHS Trust.

Eckstein, R., Wallenstein, R.S. (1958). *The Teaching and Learning of Psychotherapy.* New York: Basic Books.

International Confederation of Midwives (1993). *International Code of Ethics for Midwives.* London: ICM.

Jenkins, R. (1995). *The Law and the Midwife.* Oxford: Blackwell.

Judge, G. (1996). 'Power to the people' *The Guardian* May 11, pp.2-3.

McDowell, J. (1993). *Statutory Supervision of Midwives - in the Hands of Midwifery Managers.* unpublished MSc Dissertation, Loughborough University.

Mair, J.M.M. (1977). 'The community of self' in Bannister, D. (Ed). *New Perspectives in Personal Construct Psychology.* London: Academic Press.

Page, S. (1995). 'Letter'. *Midwives* Vol. 108, No.1, pp.228-9.

UKCC (1996). *Position Statement on Clinical Supervision for Nursing and Health Visiting.* London: UKCC.

Warwick, C. (1996). 'Leadership in midwifery care' *British Journal of Midwifery* Vol.4, No.5, p.229.

History

CHAPTER ONE

Reassessing the Guilty: The Midwives Act and the Control of English Midwives in the Early 20th Century

Brooke V. Heagerty
holds a doctorate in history from Michigan State University, with a speciality in the history of midwifery and obstetrics. The article published here draws on documents previously unavailable to researchers and revises many of the traditional tenets of British midwifery history.

The Midwives Act of 1902 created a powerful instrument for the supervision and control of midwives' practice. After 1902, no midwife could 'advertise or call herself a midwife' without registering with the state. The regulatory arm of the Act, the Central Midwives Board, redefined and restricted the scope of registered midwives' practice, formulated a course of training which prepared midwives to conform to this limited scope and created a powerful supervisory apparatus by which to enforce these restrictions. All registered midwives, regardless of training, who did not conform to these new stipulations would lose their ability to legally practice midwifery (U.K., Laws, 1902).

An 'aristocracy of midwives'

Midwifery attendance as a cause for social reform was taken up in the 1880s by the members of the small but socially well-placed Midwives Institute. For the Institute, midwifery reform was inseparable from the demand for respectable employment for middle class women and the view that the working class had to conform to the values and behaviours considered appropriate for them by their social betters. The Institute's efforts to make training and licensing mandatory for any woman who practised midwifery converged with the growing concerns over the social and economic effects of poverty and ill-health among the working class and helped to produce, with the support of their social connections and supporters within Parliament and the medical profession, the Midwives Act of 1902.

13

The Institute's early membership was largely drawn from the elite of the health professions and philanthropic work. Two of the original founders were matrons of two of London's largest lying-in hospitals. Some of the more prestigious names in the medical profession at the time, as well as the names of three members of Parliament, appear on the original Articles of Association. The leadership, the core of younger women who went on to control the policies and administration of the Institute, were all well-educated, middle and upper class women who had risen to managerial positions in obstetric wards, maternity institutions and philanthropic organizations. Through their professional life and social station, the leadership was connected to a broad network of reform-minded professionals and social activists with whom they shared a common set of values, vision and outlook for the future ('A Short History', 1933, pp.112-115; Lewis, 1994, pp.50-54; Rivers, 1981, pp.23-25; Cowell and Wainwright, 1981, pp.16-18).

The leadership sought to make midwifery into an independent profession for educated women but, as Jean Donnison has shown, they had no intention of challenging the authority of the medical profession (1977). She accurately interprets this as a tactic to gain medical consultants' support for the cause of registration, but it was by no means mere opportunism. Most of the Institute leaders were trained nurses who during their formative years had come under the influence of Florence Nightingale's nursing philosophy of which 'strict obedience to the physician's or surgeon's power and knowledge' was the first and lasting hallmark (Nightingale, 1882, p.107). Articles in the Institute's journal 'Nursing Notes' frequently sought to instil these tenets of nursing training in the practising midwife, advising her to 'uphold the doctor's authority... and do what she is told, and not either to give, or try to carry out, her own opinions' (L.B., 1900, p.156; Paget, 1901). For the Institute, the physician was the midwife's superior and the medical profession her natural ally.

The chief obstacle to the leadership's goals was not the predominantly male medical profession, but the domination of midwifery by working class lay midwives. The Institute had little firsthand knowledge of lay midwives or the lives of working class families. What they did know was filtered through the lenses of their own class and cultural perceptions. What they and other social reformers believed they saw was that irresponsibility and immorality were the prime culprits in the deteriorating conditions of working class life and that it was particularly the working class mother's ignorance of the proper values that condemned working class children to an early grave and corrupted the working class family at its heart (Lewis, 1991, pp.36-39, pp.165-167; Lewis, 1980, pp.61-87). This appeared all the more serious in light of growing fears over Britain's weakness in the face of serious economic competition from other industrializing nations (most particularly, Germany and the United States). A population racked by poverty and ill-health was hardly adequate to either defend the Empire or to labour productively for the British economy (Davin, 1978; Stedman Jones, 1971). Only through self-reliance and strict conformity to the moral code of bourgeois respectability could the working class mother rescue herself and her family from the chaos of working class life and stabilize the working class family as an essential link in the chain of social order ('The Educative', 1915, p.240; 'Practising Midwife', 1912, p.12; Chinn, 1995, pp.114-121). With other social reformers of their class, the Institute leadership believed these values were essentially alien to working class culture and that if working class women were to assimilate them, they needed the supervision of those with superior social backgrounds and refined sensibilities to do it (Heagerty, 1990, pp.42-50; 'The Nurse', 1906, p.173; 'Letting In', 1913, p.243).

The leadership's view of lay midwives was shaped not by real life midwives, but by one from fiction - Sairey Gamp, a character in Charles Dickens' novel *Martin Chuzzlewit*. For midwifery reformers, the 'Gamp' was synonymous with drunkenness, filth, carelessness with the patient, pride in ignorance and defiance of authority, and hung like a shadow over every attempt to make midwifery a profession for educated women. Her lack of formal training and her lowly class background made the 'Gamp' unfit to either attend women in childbirth or to be left with the responsibility for their moral education. Midwifery reformers believed such a woman could never 'exert a wholesome influence over her patients'. Only an educated woman and trained midwife could 'raise and refine their feelings and make them see the benefit of cleanliness and order' ('nt' 1890, p.27).

'Gamp' or not (and evidence shows that most were not), politicians recognized that if lay midwives were not allowed to practice, the country would be bereft of maternity attendants the minute the Act was signed into law. Only a small minority of midwives had any kind of formal training (the most widely acknowledged being the LOS, the diploma of the London Obstetrical Society), and the overwhelming majority of these women worked either in voluntary or Poor Law hospitals or attended wealthy women in conjunction with a physician (McCleary, 1935, p.133). It was lay midwives, working in every village, neighbourhood and town, who attended the majority of births at the turn of the century as safely, researchers have shown, as the average general practitioner at the time and under certain conditions even more so (Chamberlain, 1981, pp.112-115; Little, 1983; Wertz, 1979, pp.120-127). To guarantee an adequate number of practising midwives, the Act allowed for a grace period in which lay midwives could be registered as 'bona fide' midwives and would have their names entered on the Midwives Roll in equal standing with formally trained midwives. Lay midwives who did not register could still attend births but could not call themselves midwives and after 1910, they could no longer attend births 'habitually and for gain' without being under the immediate direction of a registered midwife or physician. That lay midwives were able to register on equal terms with the trained midwife was for the Institute leadership the only blemish on an otherwise favourable outcome. A trained midwife from Rotherham captured this sentiment when she wrote to 'Nursing Notes': 'It is an insult they should have the same status' ('Midwife', 1909, p.71).

Discipline and punish

The Act established the legal framework to govern the regulation and control of midwives' practice, but it was the Central Midwives Board (CMB) that formulated the fundamental principles upon which midwifery training, practice and supervision would be conducted. Representation on the CMB was granted to the government and to professional organizations, including the Midwives Institute, which had a vested interest in midwife regulation. Together, this elite drawn from medicine, nursing, midwifery and government service developed the principles upon which the rank and file of midwifery would carry out their work.

From its very inception, the philosophy and direction of the Central Midwives Board expressed the alliance between the medical profession and midwifery reformers. This was clearly reflected in the Rules of Practice designed by the CMB which, in Board Chairman Francis Champneys' words, put midwives 'under proper restraint' and 'in proper relation to the medical profession' (Champneys, 1908). As a means of guaranteeing the safety of midwives' practice, the Rules set out highly specific and extremely detailed requirements in the use of antiseptics and the calling of medical aid in the event of complications. But other interests were also woven into the Rules' design. By strictly limiting the scope of the midwife's practice, the Rules prevented the midwife from encroaching on the physician's territory. As she was bound to call him in the event of any complication, she served as a ready conduit to the working class obstetrical market. Further, dismantling the 'close barriers [which] are firmly erected and closely guarded by the poor', was a defining element of the Rules and an essential prerequisite of the Act's full implementation ('Book Notes', 1905, p.179). The midwife was no longer to answer to the wishes of the working class mother and her family, but to the requirements of the Rules and the middle and upper class hierarchy of the supervisory apparatus. She was expected to conform to bourgeois moral and cultural standards rather than those of the working class community in which most midwives had their roots. The Rules would force midwives to either conform or be driven from practice. If the latter, so much the better, as they would soon be replaced, midwifery reformers believed, by midwives trained with the proper understanding of their relation to the patient and to the hierarchy of authority (Heagerty, 1990, pp.50-56; 'Vacancies', 1914, p.206).

The imposition of this regime was neither a simple nor a straightforward process. The Board had to fight to impose its criteria of quality and appropriate behaviour. Enforcing the Act brought officials into direct conflict with the traditions of working class midwifery and the intricate network of working class relationships, of which the one between the midwife and the family was one of the most important. From the neighbourhood street and village road to the London offices of the CMB, the clash of different expectations, values and life experience of officials and midwives and the women they attended shaped and gave direction to the process of supervision and discipline.

'Such good friends the lot of them'

Midwifery reformers' descriptions of the trained midwife and her opposite, the Gamp, are staples of midwifery history. Yet the evidence indicates that neither were accurate readings of the composition or the characteristics of the women they were purported to describe. The relationship between the vast majority of rank and file midwives - trained and bona fide - and the women they attended was moulded by their experience as working class women, wives and mothers. It was rooted in the most fundamental and most powerful of human events, childbirth, and was strengthened by years of close association, common travails and shared social rituals (Heagerty, 1990, pp.60-72; Ross, 1983; Chinn, 1988, pp.130-147; Benson, 1989, pp.126-133). Over the years, these midwives attended many labours and knew the women they attended throughout their lives. Midwives would often stop and talk in the street with the women they attended to inquire after the baby or about the woman's health. Or they would stop and pay a 'friendly visit' to see how the family was getting along (UK Central Midwives Board, Penal Committee, 045; 028; 067; 005; 015; 038; 011; 044; 057)[1]. 'She used to have these midwives come', one woman recalled speaking of her mother, 'and they were such good friends the lot of them' (Roberts, 1984, p.107). Both trained and bona fide midwives were known to risk the loss of their certificates or lay themselves open to criminal prosecution to help the women they attended. It was not uncommon for trained and bona fide midwives alike to 'act out of sympathy with the parents' and falsify insurance notifications so that families could claim a higher benefit or to cover up abortions gone wrong so as not to involve the authorities ('Central', 1916, p.160; 'Central', 1915, p.176; 'Central', 1910, p.16; 'Central', 1911, p.6; 'Central', 1914, p.6; 'Central', 1917, p.120; 047; 063; 072; 062; 066; 019). A midwife was appreciated who did not judge, but accepted the woman and her family for what they were. 'i do not like... to be treated as a pauper if I am poor', one woman wrote to the Board in the defence of her midwife. 'i have had Mrs M- this last five times and have always been quite satisfied with her and if i have any more i do not want any body else, only Mrs M- to attend me' (048). This relationship between rank and file midwives and the women they attended represented a resilient and formidable bulwark against attempts by middle class social reformers to influence and shape working class health, culture and personal life.

This mutual respect and affection was laudable, but was this offered at the expense of quality midwifery care? Such images as that of the Staffordshire midwife who was found 'engaged in killing a pig', or Mary Ann Pickering who was convicted of being an 'abortionmonger' and sentenced to penal servitude, or Emma Jones who had to be 'picked up from a flower bed in the garden hopelessly drunk' offended refined sensibilities and provided fruitful support for midwifery reformers' position ('Rural Midwives', 1905, p.83; 'Penal Cases', 1906, p.85; 'Central', 1909, p.72; 'Law', 1911, p.128). Yet, annual reports from the local officials provided compelling evidence that bona fide midwives (the primary target of reformers' attacks) were capable, resourceful and in some areas delivered a safer service than the physician. 'It astonished me very often the amount of practical knowledge they possess, and the self-reliance they show', the Medical Officer for Northamptonshire reported. 'Most of them always welcome being shown and told better methods than their own' (UK Central Midwives Board, 1914, p.9). In a study she conducted in her district between 1907 and 1918, one Inspector found 'the lowest death rate among mothers attended by the very women that the Midwives Act, 1902 was passed to do away with. "How is it?", she asked. "These women were old, illiterate... points in their favour were that they had infinite patience, powers of observation, and left Nature to do her own work"' ('The Toll', 1931, p.36).

---

[1] A random sample of 73 cases (brought against 74 midwives) was drawn from a list of surviving case files of midwives who had been charged by the Penal Committee of the Central Midwives Board between 1905 and 1919. The individual case files will be referred to by number rather than name for purposes of confidentiality as required by the United Kingdom Central Council. The surviving penal files represent a little under half of the estimated 1500 cases against midwives during these years. The official correspondence, reports and testimony contained in each of the files provides insight into the dynamics of local supervision and the attitudes of the Inspectors, the relationship between the midwife and the women she attended, and between the woman and local midwifery officials as well as the midwife's place in the community. The citation in the reference list designates the assigned case number, the midwife's certification and the date she was called before the Board. In using quotations from these files I have not changed the language, the spelling or interrupted the flow of the language by using (sic). For a discussion of this source, see Heagerty, 1990, pp.284-289.

The front line of enforcement

Day-to-day supervision of registered midwives was the responsibility of the Local Supervisory Authorities (LSA), the supervisory apparatus created under the Act and operated by existing County and Borough Councils. The LSAs were required to conduct routine inspection of all midwives who had registered a notification to practice in their jurisdiction, to investigate any charges of malpractice, negligence or misconduct and to report any midwife who appeared guilty of such violations to the Central Midwives Board. LSAs were allowed to investigate any aspect of a midwife's practice, from following her on rounds, to questioning her patients, to investigating her living arrangements and her personal life. To refer a case to the Board, the Act required only that the LSA establish a prima facie case against the midwife, that is, they only had to submit evidence which 'on first appearance' proved the charges against her (Atkinson, pp.53-54; p.86). Most LSAs appointed a Midwifery Inspector to supervise registered midwives practising in their area. In the earlier years of the Act, an Inspector was often a member of the local gentry, a clergyman's daughter or a relative of the local MOH ('Summary', 1905, p.2).

Some local officials made genuine attempts to work with the midwives under their supervision, to instruct them in the principles of antisepsis and record keeping and to solve problems in ways that did not end in rancorous investigations and disciplinary hearings (UK Central Midwives Board, 1911, 1914; 'The Act' 1907, p.40). Many, however, had little experience with the true nature of the difficulties faced by midwives and the women they attended. They were often unable (or unwilling) to differentiate between the deliberate resistance of a truly dangerous and incompetent practitioner and a midwife who was trying to do her best for the women she attended within the limitations of her patients' poverty and chronic ill-health (Heagerty, 1990, pp.65-72; Davies, [1915] 1978). As a result, relationships between local officials and the midwives they supervised were characterized by friction and often outright hostility on both sides.

The midwifery and nursing journals routinely reported cases in which the personal prejudices and opinions of local officials had been the grounds for an investigation into a midwife's practice, for charges to be made against her, and for the Board to revoke her certificate ('The Local Authority', 1909, pp.177-178; 'The Truth', 1909, p.160). In some cases, midwives discovered that they had been cited and judged without being notified of the charges against them - a violation of the Board's own Rules (Roodhouse, 1906, p.102). It was increasingly understood that a woman did not have to fit the image of the Gamp to be vulnerable to mistreatment at the hands of the supervisory apparatus. 'I have not the courage to start as a midwife', wrote a general trained nurse who had once thought of taking up midwifery, 'I should always be afraid I should do something wrong and be hauled before the Board' ('Correspondence', 1912, p.27).

The reports filed with the CMB by Midwifery Inspectors from around the country reveal that often they evaluated midwives as much by their own criteria as by the dictates of the Rules. 'There is obviously some attempt to keep the house fairly clean', the Inspector wrote of one midwife, 'but Mrs G- lacks method' (031). They were often patronizing and judgmental. Elizabeth Harris was characterized as 'being sober and hard-working, but too ignorant and stubborn to improve by instruction' ('The Central',

1917, p.34). Inspector Hardy described Catherine Seabury as 'dirty and hopelessly ignorant' ('Penal Session', 1915, p.70). Not surprisingly, their reports often registered frustration with their work, blaming the midwife for their lack of success. Inspector Merry Smith (an Institute member) described Elizabeth Patillo as 'deaf and unintelligent; [Smith] had given her instructions... but she seemed unable to carry them out' ('Penal Cases', 1906, p.85). Some Inspectors used intimidation and harassment as a means of ridding the local authority of a midwife who had been judged troublesome. In one case the inspector 'came herself', the midwife complained to the Board, 'and urged me to resign saying I would be struck off if I did not do so'. Miss B-, the Inspector and a prominent member of the Midwives Institute, confirmed the midwife's charge, admitting, 'I am most anxious to get rid of her' (048).

As older, married women with years of experience in practice, rank and file midwives were often resentful of Inspectors' attitudes toward them. 'Many a midwife can teach a County Superintendent a good deal, is more experienced, and has attended a far greater number of cases', one midwife observed in the 'Nursing Mirror' ('Dirty Midwives', 1909, p.32). Some doubted that their inspectors, as young and as inexperienced as they sometimes were, were even competent to supervise them. Sarah Jackson, a midwife from Lancashire complained to the Board that she 'failed to understand why single, young persons should be appointed inspectors of midwives; they should in her opinion, be married, with children, then they would know as much as she did, instead of which they only knew what they read in a book' ('Penal Sessions', 1912, p.131).

A presumption of guilt permeated local officials' investigation of midwives suspected of wrongdoing. The difficulties they had in building cases against the midwives only hardened their attitude. Midwives admitted responsibility in these investigations only when they felt they had committed some wrong. Families displayed a marked reluctance to cooperate with authorities against their midwife and, like the woman described by one Town Clerk who 'whenever the Midwifery Inspector called has been most abusive', openly resisted any attempt to make them do so (022). Indeed, families were known to go to considerable lengths to defend their midwives, submitting testimonials and petitions on their behalf. The 200 names collected door to door on behalf of Mrs E - an LOS midwife, the names of 300 families living on 22 streets collected on behalf of Mrs H - or the 3000 names and attached testimonials of Mrs Pittman, a bona fide midwife from Somerset, were not unusual (065; 033; 'Central Midwives Board', 1909, p.140).

Faced with uncooperative witnesses and without the legal power to subpoena them, local officials resorted to pressure and intimidation to make their case. An Inspector might visit a woman and her family repeatedly. If this failed to work, she might take the woman to the LSA office in hopes that such surroundings would change her mind (065; 038). One County Clerk reported that 'after considerable trouble being met with direct refusal in the first instance', he had ultimately been successful, and 'Mrs T- had made an affidavit herein' (004). Other times these tactics did not work and local officials were forced to rely solely upon discrediting the midwife's character and that of her witnesses (045; 052; 002).

Midwives did not, however, simply accept the treatment meted out to them by local officials. When they felt themselves harassed or unjustly accused, they had few reservations about challenging the authority of the Act's officials. Some responded like Fanny Emory, who was reported for being, 'abusive and resentful to [her] inspector' ('Penal Session', 1913, p.12). Others merely refused to cooperate. Mrs F- was called to the town hall twice for a preliminary hearing with local officials. In neither instance was the matter resolved. Believing that she had been falsely accused in the first place, she wrote, 'I purposely kept out of employment to attend but I cannot afford to do so any longer... and I refuse to go again' (027).

'In the manner of a policeman'

While only a minority of midwives ever actually found themselves face to face with the highly educated, cultured elite of midwifery, nursing, medicine and government service that comprised the CMB, being called before the Board was an experience widely regarded with resentment and dread throughout the rank and file community. Midwives complained that rather than a forum for professional equals, the Board hearings were conducted, as one midwife described, more in 'a manner of a policeman speaking to a prisoner and not a very polite policeman at that' ('Midwives', 1912, p.361). Board chairman and obstetrician Frances Champneys' public statements give credence to midwives' complaints. For every 'conceited and reckless midwife who is too proud to advise medical help', he told his audience at the 1915 Annual Association of Inspectors meeting, 'there are ten too stupid to be able to realize what failure to attend strictly to the Rules really entails, and whose main defect is absence of imagination and sheer stupidity' (Champneys, 1915, p.170).

The Rules granted certain rights to a midwife called to a disciplinary hearing. She was allowed to cross-examine witnesses, to make a statement on her own behalf and to bring or send a friend or solicitor to represent her. She defended herself, however, against the combined resources and expertise of the Board and the LSA. Once its solicitor had determined that the evidence warranted a hearing and the midwife had been notified of the charges against her, the Board, working with the LSA, prepared the case and underwrote all prosecution expenses, including travel and lodging for its witnesses. The Board then both prosecuted the case and ruled on the evidence. Under such circumstances, it is not surprising that guilty verdicts were rendered in the majority of cases. Any judgement against the midwife, (revocation of her certificate, censure or caution) or any record of her being called before the Board in the first place, was noted in the LSA records and, if she continued to practice, could be used against her again at any time (Atkinson, 1907, pp.64-71).

A midwife, on the other hand, was one individual and usually a poor one at that. Midwives often did not have the resources to pay for the professional preparation of their cases and, as a result, sometimes unwittingly hurt their defence by appealing to community norms rather than the standards set by the CMB. Some did enlist their 'social betters' such as physicians, clergy or the local 'lady' to write letters for them or to provide character references, which were sent in with personal testimony from their patients. Midwives often could not afford to attend their hearings and were not able to fully exercise the rights granted to them under the Act. A midwife did have the right to appeal the Board's decision in High Court, but this was an expensive procedure beyond the reach of many rank and file midwives.

The prima facie evidence presented by the LSA was the foundation for any case against a midwife. Sometimes the testimony, pattern of practice and the record of notifications clearly established the midwife's responsibility. But this was by no means the norm. Guilty judgements based on 'very conflicting evidence' and 'very little evidence', as 'Nursing Notes' put it in two cases of midwives who lost their certificates, were a common occurrence ('Penal Cases', 1911, p.178). Midwife H -, for example, was severely censured despite her good record, the fact that the family would not testify against her and that she had in fact called in a physician, even though the family had opposed it (001). The Board also employed a liberal definition of hearsay. An official's claim that the violation had occurred was often proof enough of a midwife's guilt. Midwives were disciplined solely on Inspectors' unsubstantiated claims that midwives had 'confessed' (004; 040; 060). Although both denied the charges and no other proof was offered, Midwife D - was severely censured and Midwife B - struck off on this type of evidence. Local officials hounded Midwife P - simply on a local physician's claim that he had frequently seen her drunk 'in the streets, but not at a Confinement' (002). (As the two had been competing over cases for years, he was hardly a disinterested source.) Nevertheless, like two other midwives who had no problem with their practice but had been 'rumoured to have been seen drinking', Midwife P - was struck off (063; 068).

Midwifery reformers argued that when women and children became sick or died, it was the midwife's negligence and her overweening pride in her abilities which were responsible. There were undoubtedly times in which these factors played a defining role in the outcome of midwives' cases. Other evidence suggests, however, that midwives were faced with a much more complex situation than midwifery reformers understood or would admit. Poverty, poor housing and ill-health were the realities which shaped the lives of the women who midwives attended and were therefore the contours of midwives' practice. The Rules made no allowance for these facts, yet held midwives responsible when this reality prevented the Rules full implementation. This can be seen in almost any category of charges brought by the Board, but was probably no more true than in the most common charge against midwives regardless of training: 'failure to advise and send for a physician'.

Of the cases drawn from the random sample of CMB penal files, 69 per cent were in the category of 'failure to advise and send for a physician'. In 40 per cent of these cases, the cost of the physician's services caused the family to refuse the midwife's recommendation for a physician or for the midwife to delay in sending for one. In 13 per cent of the cases, although the midwives were blamed, it was the physician who was responsible for the poor outcome of the case. In 18 per cent of the cases, the midwife had not even failed to call a physician, but rather had been accused of failing to submit notification to the LSA. Only the remaining 15 cases out of the 51 (29 per cent) involved questions of the midwife's compliance with the requirement to send for a physician in the event of complications (not all of which were proved conclusively). Eighty-six per cent of midwives in the sample charged under this category were found guilty. Fifty-three per cent were struck off and 33 per cent were either censured or cautioned. Trained and bona fide midwives were struck off in roughly equal percentages, 54 per cent and 58 per cent respectively.

The Rules did not require a midwife to get the physician herself, but she did have to inform the family and hand to them the official form notifying that she was advising and sending for medical aid. If they were poor, families were often reluctant to act on her advice even if the midwife insisted. This put the midwife in an extremely difficult position, 'standing as she did between the Rules laid down by the CMB and the urgent desire for delay on the patient's part' ('Local Government', 1907, p.157). Midwife S - advised for the doctor 'and the people promised to send for one', wrote one local doctor on her behalf. 'No doubt their extreme poverty… delayed their doing so' (020; 055; 052; 012; 001). In some cases, midwives made the decision themselves because of their knowledge of the family. One midwife did not 'see the necessity of sending for a doctor' in the death of a premature infant 'as the patient was very poor' (001).

Midwives were also disciplined for poor outcomes when it was actually the physician they had called who was responsible. Physicians' refusal to respond to a midwife's call for help and physicians' misdiagnosis were the two most common forms of this. Fear of losing out on a fee was often cited as the reason doctors would not attend a case, or, as some suspected, retribution for the competition a midwife presented to his practice. 'It is dreadful to have to send to two or three before one will come', one midwife recounted. In one of her cases, 'the husband went for eight doctors, but could not get one. I went round to [one] and begged him to come' ('The Payment', 1908, p.66). Technically, the Rules protected a midwife when this occurred (Atkinson, 1907, p.79), but there were cases in which the Board held midwives responsible nevertheless. Midwife R-, for example, called the physician the day of the birth, but he did not come until almost 24 hours later (064). The physician Midwife F- summoned did not come until three hours after he had been requested (027). The infants concerned, eventually diagnosed with opthalmia neonatorum, suffered permanent damage to their eyes. Both Mrs R- and Mrs F- were struck off.

Yet midwives' problems did not necessarily end when the physician arrived. Midwives L- and C- finding a rise in temperature, fetched the doctor. 'He examined the patient', the Inspector's report recounted, 'and told the midwife it was not Sepsis but the excitement that had upset the girl' (025). The woman died. The doctor called in by Midwife B - in a case of suspected abortion signed a declaration that he did not know how to treat the woman, believing that 'a supper of fried eels on Saturday evening' had caused her symptoms (062). Of the seven cases in the sample of this type, five resulted in death. While it appears the physicians were not even reprimanded, the midwives involved suffered heavy penalties. Four of the midwives were struck off, two were severely censured and two were cautioned.

The Board was not about to enter into the business of judging the ethics of medical practitioners or the quality of their practice. Neither were they interested in the wishes of the families midwives attended. The intention of the Rules was to remove, as much as possible, discretionary power from the midwife's hands and to force her to behave in keeping with the professional and personal standards set out by the Board (Atkinson, 1907 p.72). A 'good' midwife did not question this (or anything else), but followed the Rules to the letter regardless of the consequences to others. 'The Rules of the Board were to be obeyed', Champneys told one midwife before the Board, 'whether a midwife liked them or not; and the superior officers were there to be obeyed whether a midwife liked them or not' ('Penal Board', 1916, p.92; 'Penal Board', 1914, p.18).

If a midwife expressed deference to the Board and to the authority of her supervisors, she was more likely to keep her certificate, regardless of the severity of their actions. Despite the fact that a child had gone blind under her care, the Board, due to the fact that 'she had acknowledged her error, and in consideration of her good character' decided 'not to strike her off the Roll, but to censure her severely' ('Central Midwives Board', 1912, p.196). If she refused, she was treated like Ellen Kerens, to whom Champneys replied, that 'before re-admission to the roll she would have to prove, not only that she realized the enormity of her action, but of her own attitude toward it' ('Penal Board', 1917, p.34).

The Board considered it as important for a midwife to 'go through life wearing the white flower of a blameless life' (Moberly, 1900, p.132) as it was for her to show deference and submission to social and professional superiors. Before a woman was allowed to register as a midwife, she had to provide verification of her 'good character' (Atkinson, 1907, p.60). Failure to live up to this standard not only brought the entire profession into disrepute but jeopardized, in midwifery reformers' minds, the crusade against the poverty and ill-health which threatened the foundations of British society and the power of the Empire around the world. In such cases, as in consideration of her 'attitude', the Board did not concern itself with the midwife's abilities or the record of her practice, but rather her 'character', that is her behaviour, her values, her comportment in daily life (Heagerty, 1990, 50-56; 94; 'Penal Board', 1916, p.200). Moral lapses such as out-of-wedlock children, extramarital affairs, and drinking whether on or off duty occurred among both trained and bona fide midwives and were almost always grounds for automatically losing one's certificate.

Not surprisingly, the Board extended greater sympathy and respect to women whose class background or whose social connections were similar to those of its members. This could be expressed in seemingly minor favours such as withholding the names of two midwives 'removed from the Roll for lapses from the moral code; they both held the CMB examination certificate'. At a time when many rank and file midwives' names and their transgressions were published throughout the midwifery press, for these women, 'Nursing Notes' reported, 'The Chairman requested the press withhold their names in consideration for their friends' ('Penal Proceedings', 1912, p.74). Similarly, Midwife H-, a member of the Midwives' Institute, who had mistaken puerperal fever for hysteria, did not take the woman's temperature although the Rules required it, and stated her only reason for calling the doctor being that, 'I felt I could not manage [the patient] any longer', was merely cautioned to observe the Rules. In her file was a letter from Paula Fynes-Clinton, the Honorary Secretary of the Midwives' Institute, who had written, 'It would give me great pleasure to hear that the Board has been able to judge her case leniently' (024; 'Penal Cases', 1910, p.198).

Not all midwives submitted to the Board's authority. 'If you have the right to suspend my Certificate, please enforce your right', Mrs B - wrote to the Board. 'I have practised as a midwife for 40 years and have never lost a case. So you proceed as you see fit' (050). Similarly, Mrs M- vowed to continue practising and refused to return her certificate to the Board, writing, 'Sir, I must remind you that it is my property and I paid for it' (037). Others were less vocal about their intentions, but defied the Board nevertheless. A few months after she lost her certificate, Mrs K- was fined 20 shillings in Police Court for attending a woman in childbirth (038). In 1914, Mrs P-, who had earned her LOS in

1899, was 'discovered attending births again' one year after her certificate had been revoked (055; 'Burnley', 1910, p.36; 'Gloucester', 1911, p.40; 'Still Practising', 1911, p.128; 'Defiant Midwife', 1910, p.254; 'Correspondence', 1912, p.182; 'From Far', 1911, p.40; UK Central Midwives Board, 1915, p.9).

'Women may be fairly satisfied'

The restrictions on midwives and the inequities in the Board's penal process were not as objectionable to the Institute as one might expect. The Institute leadership had achieved many of its goals through the Midwives Act: the title of midwife was protected, normal midwifery had been identified as the midwife's preserve, a recognized body, the Central Midwives Board, had been established through which midwives' training and practice was to be regulated, and the Midwives Institute had secured a seat on that governing body. The leadership had no objection to the requirement that they appoint a physician to fill their seat on the CMB and preferred to have a male consultant, rather than a midwife, to represent them ('Midwife Representation', 1907, p.103). With five of the nine Board members either Institute members or supporters, the Institute was well-placed to influence the development of the profession at the highest level and felt that 'women as women may be fairly satisfied' ('The Central Midwives Board', 1902, pp.153-154).

Moreover, the Institute was an active partner in the promulgation and imposition of the Board's philosophy of supervision and control. Through her position as the chair of the committee which 'drafted the reports and recommendations' concerning midwives' practice, for example, Rosalind Paget helped to define the limitations on midwives' work and to formulate the restrictions under which they were required to perform their designated tasks ('District Nursing', 1904, p.73). As members of the penal committee, both Rosalind Paget and Jane Wilson actively participated in the Board's disciplinary work.

For the Institute leadership, the real problem was that local authorities were making no distinction between trained and bona fide midwives in the manner of their supervision or in their recommendations to the Board. When local officials did not understand that the Rules were at once their weapon to drive bona fide midwives from practice and their tool to improve trained midwifery attendance, 'trained midwives are bound to suffer', 'Nursing Notes' protested, and 'have every right to feel themselves the victims of an *undiscriminating* legal machinery' [italics mine] ('Protection', 1911, p.295). By placing the cream of midwifery on the same level as the most 'degraded' of practitioners, local officials' actions would 'deter the very women we most want from taking up the task' and the field would be left to the women the Act was intended to supplant ('Monmouthshire', 1910, p.194). If some reform was not effected in local supervision, 'the work the CMB has done... [will] be wasted and the Act... [will] become a dead letter' ('The Delegation', 1917, p.45). Instead, the Institute believed, professionally qualified Inspectors, educated women with 'considerable practical experience... a trained nurse... who had experience in the training and supervision of subordinates' could help trained midwives improve their practice, solve problems without resorting to threats and discipline and handle the bona fide with an eye to her removal ('Inspection', 1914, p.173). This kind of approach, the Institute believed, would make the profession more attractive to educated women while at the same allowing the Act to do the work for which it was intended.

Conclusion

The formidable power the Board wielded so liberally was the key weapon in the struggle to transform midwifery from an occupation of working class women enmeshed in the working class community and trained in traditional methods to a profession of CMB trained midwives aloof from such entanglements and in step with the medical profession, the elite of midwifery and the agenda of midwifery reform.

Midwifery reformers defended the Rules' restrictions and the powers of the supervisory apparatus in the name of protecting women and children from dangerous practitioners. This should not be discounted as mere opportunism. Their commitment in this regard was no less sincere for being inseparable from their own professional self-interest and class outlook. Midwifery reformers sought to use the registered trained midwife as an instrument through which the complex of their aims could be realized - whether she was providing the moral education for the working class mother, acting as a conduit to the obstetrical market or serving as the vehicle for respectable employment for middle class women.

Rank and file resistance was not, as midwifery reformers claimed, the act of socially marginal and dangerous practitioners, but a response to the Rules' separation of mother and midwife and the punitive restrictions placed on midwives' lives and practice. Midwives' social and personal lives were interwoven with those of the women they attended. Disrupting and destroying one relationship jeopardized all the other myriad ties which connected her to her broader community. When she fought to protect this relationship (either by submitting to the family's wishes or quarrelling with local officials), she was fighting for her sense of herself as a midwife. It was this sense of self which the Board ultimately had to break if it was to achieve its aims. While the Board may have succeeded in reconfiguring the outward structures of midwives lives and practice, destroying this inner sense of what it means to be a midwife has proven to be a far more complicated and lengthy process than reformers ever imagined.

References

'A Short History of the Institute' (1933). *Nursing Notes* August, pp.112-115.

Atkinson, S. (1907). *The Office of Midwife in England and Wales*. London: Bailliere, Tindall and Cox.

Benson, J. (1989). *The Working Class in Britain, 1850-1939*. London: Longman.

'Book Notes' (1905). *Nursing Notes* December p.179.

Brierly, E. (1923). 'In the beginning'. *Nursing Notes* January pp.9-10.

'Burnley' (1910). *Nursing Notes* February p.36.

'Central Midwives Board' (1909). *Nursing Notes* July p.140.

'Central Midwives Board' [Maria Penfold] (1910). *Nursing Notes* January p.16.

'Central Midwives Board' (1911). *Nursing Notes* August p.201.

'Central Midwives Board' [Sarah Dean] (1911). *Nursing Notes* January p.16.

'Central Midwives Board' [Jane Harvey] (1914). *Nursing Notes* January p.16.

'Central Midwives Board' [Charlotte Elizabeth Downsell] (1915). *Nursing Notes* July p.176.

'Central Midwives Board' [Mary Ann Southern] (1912). *Nursing Notes* July p.196.

'Central Midwives Board' [Ethel Irwin] (1916). *Nursing Notes* July p.160.

'Central Midwives Board' [Alice Louise Roadnight, CMB certified] (1917). *Nursing Notes* July p.120.

Chamberlain, M. (1981). *Old Wives Tales*. London: Virago.

Champneys, F. (1908). 'Midwives in England'. *St. Bartholomew's Hospital Journal.* Vol. XV.

'Address delivered to the Association of Inspectors of Midwives'. *Nursing Notes* July, pp.169-170. 1915.

Chinn, C. (1995). *Poverty Admist Prosperity: the Urban Poor in England, 1834-1914.* New York: St. Martins Press.

They Worked All Their Lives: Women of the Urban Poor in England,1860-1939. Manchester: Manchester University Press. 1988.

'Correspondence' (1912). *Nursing Notes* October p.182.

'Correspondence' (1912). *Nursing Notes* January p.27.

Cowell, B., D, Wainwright. (1981). *Behind the Blue Door: The History of the Royal College of Midwives 1881-1981.* London: Bailliere Tindall.

Davin, A. (1978). 'Imperialism and motherhood'. *History Workshop Journal.* 5. Spring pp.9-65.

Davies, M. L. (1978). *Maternity: Letters from Working Women..* London: Bell and Sons. 1915. Reprint. New York: W.W. Norton & Company.

'Defiant midwife' (1910). *Nursing Notes* October p.254.

'Dirty midwives' (1909). *Nursing Mirror* September 18 p.32.

'District nursing notes' (1904). *Nursing Notes* May p.73.

Donnison, J. (1977). *Midwives and Medical Men.* New York: Schocken Books.

French, M. (1915). 'The Educative influence of the midwife' *Nursing Notes* October p.240.

'From far and near'. (1911). *Nursing Notes* February p.40.

'Gloucester' (1911). *Nursing Notes* February p.40.

Heagerty, B. V. (1990). *Class, Gender and Professionalization: The Struggle for British Midwifery, 1900-1936.* Ph.D. diss. Michigan State University.

'Inspection from the midwives point of view' (1914). *Nursing Notes* June pp.173-174.

L.B. (1900). 'Nursing notes for practical nurses'. *Nursing Notes* November pp.155-156.

'Law and police' (1911). *Nursing Notes* May p.128.

'Letting in the light' (1913). *Nursing Notes* September p.243.

Lewis, J. (1980). *The Politics of Motherhood: Child and Maternal Welfare in England 1900-1939.* London: Croom Helm.

Lewis, J. (1991). *Women and Social Action in Victorian and Edwardian England.* Stanford: Stanford University Press.

Lewis, J. (1994). 'Gender, the family and women's agency in the building of welfare states: the British case'. *Social History,* Vol.19, No.1. pp.37-55.

Little, B. (1983). *Go Seek Mrs. Dawson. She'll know what to do - The Demise of the Working Class Nurse/Midwife in the Twentieth Century.* Unpublished Thesis. University of Sussex. Duplicated.

'Local government board circular: medical aid' (1907). *Nursing Notes,* October p.157.

McCleary, G. F. (1935). *The Maternity and Child Welfare Movement.* London: P. S. King & Son.

'Midwife Notes' (1909). *Nursing Notes* April pp.71-72.

'Midwife representation' (1907). *Nursing Notes* July p.103.

'Midwives before the CMB' (1912). *Nursing Times.* April 6 p.361.

Moberly, L.G. (1900). 'Private Nurses'. *Nursing Notes* September p.132.

Nightingale, F. (1882). 'Training of nurses and nursing the sick poor', reprinted from Dr. Quain. *Dictionary of Medicine.* Quoted in Gamarnikow, E. (1978). 'Sexual division of labour: The case of nursing' in Kuhn, A., Wolpe, A.M. *Feminism and Materialism.* London: Routledge.

'nt' (1890). *Nursing Notes* March p.27.

Paget, R. (1901). *Letter to John Dakin.* February. Royal College of Midwives Archives, London.

'Penal Board' (1916). *Nursing Notes* July p.160.

'Penal Board [Agnes Sarah Quinton]' (1916). *Nursing Notes* April p.92.

'Penal Board [Elizabeth Morgans]' (1916). *Nursing Notes* September p.200.

'Penal Cases' (1906). *Nursing Notes* June p.85.

'Penal Cases [Mary Jane Barrett]' (1910). *Nursing Notes* August p.198.

'Penal Cases [Anna Hooper; Mary Ann Spate]' (1911). *Nursing Notes* July p.178.

'Penal Cases [Emilie Victoria Pocock]' (1914). *Nursing Notes* January p.18.

'Penal Proceedings' (1912). *Nursing Notes* March p.74.

'Penal Session' (1913). *Nursing Notes* January p.12.

'Penal Session' (1915). *Nursing Notes* March p.70.

'Penal Sessions' (1912). *Nursing Notes* May p.131.

'Practising Midwife: The influence of the midwife' (1912) *Nursing Notes* January p.12.

Rivers, J. (1981). *Dame Rosalind Paget. A Short Account of her Life and Work.* London: Midwives Chronicle.

Roberts, E. (1984). *A Woman's Place.* Oxford: Basil Blackwell.

Roodhouse, A.M. (1906). '?' *Nursing Notes* July p.102.

Ross, E. (1983). 'Survival networks: women's neighborhood sharing in London before World War I'. *History Workshop Journal*, 15, pp.4-27.

Rules Framed By the Central Midwives Board Under the Midwives Act of 1902 and 1919. (1919). London: Spottiswoode, Ballantyne & Co.

'Rural Midwives Association' (1905). *Nursing Notes* June p.83.

Stedman-Jones, G. (1971). *Outcast London.* Oxford: Oxford University Press.

'Still Practising Though Removed from the Roll' (1911). *Nursing Notes* May p.128.

'Summary of Work, 1904: The Midwives Act' (1905). *Nursing Notes* January pp.2-3.

'The Act in the Country' (1907). *Nursing Notes* March p.40.

'The Central Midwives Board' (1917). *Nursing Notes* February p.34.

'The Delegation of the Inspection of Midwives' (1917). *Nursing Notes* March pp.45-46.

'The Local Authority and the Midwife' (1909). *Nursing Notes* September pp.177-178.

'The Monmouthshire Training Home' (1910). *Nursing Notes* August p.194.

'The Nurse and the Midwife as Citizens' (1906). *Nursing Notes* December pp.173-174.

'The Payment of Doctors' Cases' (1908). *Nursing Notes* March p.66.

'The Penal Board' (1917). *Nursing Notes.* February pp.34-35.

'The Protection of the Midwife' (1911). *Nursing Notes* December pp.295-296.

'The Toll of Motherhood' (1931). *Nursing Notes.* March p.36.

'The Truth of the Matter' (1909). *Nursing Notes* August p.160.

'Vacancies for certified midwives' (1914). *Nursing Notes.* July p.206.

Wertz, R. W., Wertz, D.C. (1979). *Lying-In. A History of Childbirth in America.* New York: Schocken Books.

Government documents

United Kingdom Laws, Statutes, etc. (1902). *Midwives Act, 1902* 2 Edw. 7 Ch. 17.

United Kingdom Central Midwives Board (1911). *The Work of the Board Ending March 1911.* Royal College of Midwives Archives, London.

United Kingdom Central Midwives Board (1914). *The Work of the Board Ending March 1914.* Royal College of Midwives Archives, London.

United Kingdom Central Midwives Board (1915). *The Work of the Board Ending March 1915.* Royal College of Midwives Archives, London.

United Kingdom Public Record Office, Central Midwives Board. (1905 – 1910). Penal Committee.

Case files of the Central Midwives Board Penal Committee cited by author's #, training, year of disciplinary hearing:

001. BF. 1917.	024. BF. 1915.	045. BF. 1918.	064. LOS. 1919.
002. BF. 1906.	025. CMB. 1918.	047. BF. 1919.	065. LOS. 1919
004. BF. 1908.	027. CMB. 1916	048. BF. 1919.	066. Salvation Army.
005. BF. 1909.	028. CMB. 1915.	050. BF. 1919.	1908.
011. CMB. 1911.	031. CMB. 1917	052. LOS. 1908.	067. Manchester
012. BF. 1912	033. BF. 1918.	055. LOS. 1913	Maternity. 1909.
015. BF. 1912	037. BF. 1917.	057. LOS. 1915.	068. Trained nurse and
019. BF. 1914	038. BF. 1917.	060. LOS. 1917.	trained midwife,
020. BF. 1914	040. BF, 1918.	062. LOS. 1918.	1909.
022. CMB. 1915.	044. BF. 1918.	063. BF. 1918.	072. CMB. 1916

CHAPTER TWO

Supervision of Midwives in Nottingham 1948-72

Julia Allison MA, RM, ADM, Cert Ed (FE) (Dist) MTD
worked as a community midwife for 16 years in Nottinghamshire and became a midwifery adviser to the Nottingham Health Authority before going to be Head of the Faculty of Midwifery at Norfolk and Norwich College of Nursing. Mrs Allison has completed her PhD research into home births, looking at the records of district midwives in Nottingham between 1948 and 1974, wanting her research to demonstrate the safety of home births. Her career has culminated in her becoming General Secretary of the Royal College of Midwives in March 1994.

Mavis Kirkham RGN, RM, BA, MA, PhD, Cert Ed (Adult), FP Nursing Cert
is currently Professor of Midwifery at the University of Sheffield. She has 20 years of experience of clinical midwifery and research and five years of midwifery education

As time has passed some of the factors separating Inspectors and midwives have changed and the gap between them narrowed. The payment by the local authority to GPs (1918) when called by a midwife helped poor families, eased their midwives' dilemmas and improved the midwife's chances of getting paid for cases also attended by a GP. Monetary compensation (1926) for midwives suspended from practice after contact with infection also helped poor midwives and their families.

The 1936 Midwives Act required Local Supervising Authorities (LSAs) to provide a salaried midwifery service. From this point supervision and management, whilst separate functions in law, were potentially difficult to separate in practice.

The 1937 Ministry of Health Letter is significant in that it acknowledged many of the problems being experienced with supervision and sought to remedy them. The Letter acknowledged the 'bad psychological effect upon the midwife' of being supervised by someone without knowledge of midwifery. Supervisors were therefore required to have 'adequate experience in the practice of midwifery'. The Letter stated that an Inspector of Midwives should be regarded as the 'counsellor and friend of the midwife, rather than as a relentless critic'. She should have 'sympathy and tact' and be called a supervisor rather than an inspector.

The structure of supervision: Nottingham 1948-72

This chapter examines the supervision of midwives over a 24 year period from the implementation of the National Health Service (NHS) in 1948 up to its reorganization in 1972. It is based upon historical research into district midwifery in Nottingham during that time. Supervision is only one part of that study (Allison, 1996).

Between 1948 and 1972 local authorities provided domiciliary midwifery services for up to 50 per cent of births which took place at home. The system changed over time as a consequence of local government reforms (HMSO, 1969) and the recommendations of Cranbrook (HMSO, 1959) and Peel (HMSO, 1970) for increased numbers of women to be 'confined' in hospital. It was finally abandoned at the reorganization of the NHS (HMSO, 1972), although the demise of an effective domiciliary midwifery service was more to do with the assumption that birth in hospital was safest for all women.

There was a national shortage of midwives throughout most of this period and the district midwives of Nottingham carried an average caseload of 100 cases per year: almost double that recommended by the 1949 government working party. District midwives were appointed by the Medical Officer of Health (MOH). They were appointed as midwifery sisters and worked as individual practitioners in a non hierarchical service, giving caseload care to their own clients and liaising in partnerships to provide reciprocal cover for their clients. District midwives lived within and had responsibility for their own 'patch'. They provided continuity of care for women booked for home birth and all social and domestic aspects of birth were the province of the district midwife whatever the place of birth.

The district midwives interviewed could see no similarity between present day team midwifery and the way in which they worked. They saw themselves, though salaried, as working independently in that they had their own caseload of women for whom they had total responsibility. They recognized their responsibility to the supervisor of midwives but did not see her as their manager. Indeed supervisors continued to work clinically covering wherever relief was needed. In particular the midwives' clinics were regularly and frequently covered by the supervisor when the midwife was at a labour call or sleeping after attending labours at night. In this sense supervisors fitted into the system as colleagues and helpers rather than as managers.

Supervision of midwives was carried out by the local health authority, acting as the LSA, and exercised by the MOH or any person appointed by him for the purpose. As the Medical supervisor of midwives throughout this period was the MOH, whose range of responsibilities included housing, education and social services, the supervision of midwives was undertaken within the overall context of women's lives and the relevant public health issues.

The MOH was responsible for the annual publication of birth statistics and maternity outcomes. Changing social circumstances and professional developments were acknowledged by increased data collection, e.g. in the 1950s the MOH began to identify mothers by their country of origin. In his annual report the MOH made qualitative and quantitative comparisons between years. Tables and charts were given with comparative data for home and hospital births, but no systematic or rigorous analysis was attempted. Other aspects of the health and well-being of the local population were similarly described. The fact that data was recorded and reported does not necessarily mean that it is heeded and if proper interpretation of this data had been made and presented to the Peel Committee, it would have been difficult for the argument for 100 per cent hospital births on the grounds of safety to be sustained. After the reorganization of the NHS in 1972, no systematic data collection or publication of maternity outcomes appear to have been taken which reflect the role of the midwife. Indeed the 1979 House of Commons 'Perinatal and Mortality Report' (HMSO, 1980) recommended that less birth data be recorded.

The non medical supervisors of midwives (i.e. the midwife supervisors hereafter referred to as supervisors) were required to have been in active practice as a midwife for a minimum of three years with one years district experience. They worked effectively largely because of their location in relation to the LSA and their relationships with midwives and mothers. The locus of the LSA was the local authority, housed in the public health department. The offices of the supervisors were similarly located in that department in close proximity to the MOH. They reported to him on a regular basis and worked with him in compiling midwifery data for presentation in annual reports. They did not see themselves as managed by him, in the modern sense of that word, nor did they experience managerial constraints on their supervision of midwives. Thus whilst the supervision of midwives was, at this time, grounded in the context of public health, it was also entirely composed of persons with qualification and proven expertise in maternity care. Furthermore the entire focus and location of domiciliary midwifery was district based with no functional, financial or executive control from hospital based services.

The work of the supervisor

It is clear from the work and oral evidence of the supervisors in this study that they viewed their function in terms of protecting mothers and babies. They achieved this through supervised deliveries and postnatal 'nursings' and comprehensive scrutiny of midwives' personal registers, labour notes and drug prescriptions.

Supervisors played an important role in collecting statistics of both midwives and births. The fact that they had an overview of the district midwives workload also involved them in the managerial work of endeavouring to make that workload more equitable. They tried to address this by asking midwives to keep a district register of all women booked by them for home birth to compare with the number they subsequently delivered. If there was a clear imbalance between bookings and deliveries, the supervisor would redefine geographical boundaries from time to time to redress the balance.

As the number of hospital births rose, early discharge from hospital with transfer of care to district midwives became the norm. By the late 1960s several district midwives were employed on a part-time basis to provide relief cover and assistance with postnatal care of hospital delivered women. The repetitious nature of these duties, together with the lack of opportunity for these part-time midwives to utilize their full range of skills was later to lead to a review by the supervisor who decided that all midwives, whether part-time or full-time, should carry a caseload. This decision was reached after discussion at a meeting with all district midwives and in such a way that midwives were clear as to the reasons for the supervisor's actions, which were to maintain high standards of care for mothers and of morale for midwives. The supervisor felt that midwives lost their motivation and interest when caring for women they had not delivered and with whom they had no relationship. Postnatal care therefore suffered from being performed by rota. There was also danger of a midwife with a very restricted area of practice being called to an emergency with which she might not be able to cope. As they lacked job satisfaction there was a high turnover of part-time midwives but since they were paid pro rata to the full time rate a few full time midwives opted to work part time as the part time working conditions were seen as an easier option. After the decision that all midwives should carry a caseload, up dating was planned individually for each part time midwife, in hospital and with district colleagues. The way in which this matter was resolved shows an insight into midwives' working situation which is rarely achieved in hospital practice.

Nevertheless, the supervisor of midwives in the 1940s was a figure of great authority from whom midwives and mothers still sometimes conspired to conceal issues of mutual concern.

Miss Millbank was a popular Nottingham midwife who in the later years of her service began to go blind with cataracts. In those days midwives did not get their pension unless they completed service to retirement age and Miss Millbank battled bravely on until she was too blind to ride her bike. Eventually it was discovered by her supervisor that she was attending her calls and delivering babies by pushing all her equipment from house to house in an old pram, given to her by one of the mothers. So great was the mothers' loyalty to her that no-one had complained. Finally she was retired from service a few weeks before her official retirement age. After a lot of fuss and threats to expose the Local Authority's meanness to the press she was finally paid her superannuation and pension.

It is interesting that the supervisor was clearly identified with the employing authority in the minds of those involved in this incident. She was identified as protecting mothers and babies but not as a 'counsellor and friend' to Miss Millbank.

From the oral evidence of the supervisors the following list of duties has been drawn up:

- 24 hour cover by one of the two supervisors for emergency contact by district midwives
- three monthly supervisory visits to midwives' homes for record and drug checks
- arranging off duty and 24 hour cover for all labours and emergencies in the City
- arranging placements for district pupil midwives, medical students and student nurses
- holiday rotas
- issuing prescriptions
- issuing, replacing and checking uniforms and equipment
- teaching district pupils about maternal and child health issues for an hour twice weekly

- acting as relief for clinics when midwives were attending a birth
- attending births in a supervisory capacity - sometimes with pupils
- taking parentcraft sessions
- collecting and collating data for the MOH
- report writing for the MOH.

This is how Nellie, a retired supervisor, described her day:

'In a day you dealt with midwives coming into the office for prescriptions for Pethidine... for uniforms... equipment... changing... we did a lot of paperwork for the MOH... sorting out the records that were kept. I used to attend clinics and attend parentcraft... they were all short of manpower... the birth-rate was so high... you couldn't guarantee all the midwives would be there. I kept my hand in at clinical teaching... I used to take the district pupils... I also used to do revision on midwifery aspects as well as the public health side'.

Work done by the supervisor of midwives and assistant supervisor City of Nottingham 1955

Visits to midwives and inspection of records and equipment	184
Inspection of midwives in nursing homes	11
Special domiciliary visits:	
Expectant and nursing mothers	229
Stillbirths	10
Puerperal pyrexia	32
Skin condition	14
Office interviews regarding hospital confinements	571

Table 2.1: Work done by the supervisor of midwives and assistant supervisor, Nottingham 1955.

Source: Medical Officer of Health Report, 1995.
(reproduced with permission from Allison, J. (1996). *Delivered at Home*. London: Chapman and Hall. p.31, Table 1.6)

This was clearly the workload of a highly experienced practising midwife. There was none of the separation of supervision from the realities of practice so evident at the beginning of the century (see Chapter 1). Some of this was also management work. The pattern of supervisory duties remained fairly constant until the late 1960s.

Supervisory visits to midwives' homes

Supervisory visits to district midwives' homes were an important part of supervision. District midwives worked from home and in so far as her home was her working base the midwife's house was inspected along with her records and her equipment. On the appointed day the midwife had ready her records, registers, casenotes, drug box, work diary, uniform and equipment and any locally required records. She would need to show evidence of her clinic work, attendances and follow up. Her equipment was checked, her uniform, bag linings and gowns were also inspected and counted. The place where her drugs were stored in her home was checked for security and any rooms in which she interviewed or examined women were inspected for cleanliness and appropriateness. A supervisory visit would take at least half a day to complete. All records were examined, registers and casenotes were checked against the drug records and prescriptions. Critical incidents, such as stillbirths, maternal deaths and occasions when the flying squad were called would be reflected upon. At the end of the session the supervisor would sign and date the midwife's register in red ink. The registers of City and County of Nottingham district midwives demonstrate that this task was assiduously carried out throughout the years of this study.

Supervisory visits demonstrate clearly the evolution of the supervisory role. A large element of inspection was required of supervisors at this time. Yet the registers demonstrate that midwives were supported in the individuality of their approaches to practice. The supervisors did not constrain the district midwives to write to a formula but let them keep registers in their own style, providing they were within statutory requirements. Supervisory visits also involved discussion of critical incidents and reflection on practice. After stillbirths or neonatal deaths midwives were often led to ask questions rather than being told answers. They were also advised to discuss issues with colleagues at a time when district midwives, even in a city, practiced in real isolation and knew little of each other's practice. Midwives could therefore find these supervisory visits to be a 'growing experience'.

In hundreds of hours of interviews with midwives there were no criticism of their supervisors. There were, however, numerous expressions of respect for the person and the role. Many paid tribute to the fact that the supervisor and her deputy covered every day and night of the year to ensure that there was always a supervisor on call. Several quoted incidents where, because of the insight of the supervisor, midwives who were committing misdemeanours were 'found out' before a tragedy occurred. These involved cases of pethidine abuse and midwives not performing their duties safely because of stress or mental illness. It is also a testament to the supervisor's skill and approachability that midwives frequently recognized that her wide experience in midwifery and public health made her an appropriate person to turn to when they had a 'bad social case'.

The allocation of hospital beds on social grounds

The pressure for hospital beds on social grounds constantly exceeded the number available. There were 763 applications in 1962, of which 410 were granted (City of Nottingham, 1962/26). The medical officer failed to acknowledge that 353 women who were not granted hospital beds were returned to their district midwife to be delivered in a home which had already been identified as unsuitable. Thus 11 per cent of the city's home births in 1962 tool place in home conditions which had been identified as unsuitable for home birth.

Nellie, a retired supervisor of midwives who had the thankless task of deciding to whom the beds should be allocated, shared these recollections:

> 'They used to have such things as "social beds", it was part of my job to go and vet them. The midwife used to vet them first, there wasn't any criteria really for home delivery, what it amounted to was if the mother and father had a bedroom to themselves, even if they were sharing a terraced house with another family, they were put down for a home delivery. You couldn't make demands about inside toilets and running hot water, because more didn't have it than did. We used to put them down (for a social bed) if the midwife said the house was not suitable we knew it was beyond the pale, these were usually the really dirty houses, and so we put them down for a social bed, but half didn't get one.'

In these circumstances the district midwife might negotiate with the housing department to fumigate the house, the electricity board to reconnect a disconnected supply and beg essentials from local charities or tradesmen.

It could be argued that, with such experienced district midwives who were able to ensure good outcomes of care even in home conditions identified as unsuitable, appropriate packages of care could have been targeted at those babies born in poverty which were at least as cost effective as hospital confinement. On an individual level, midwives appear to have been doing this in their own practice.

Infant feeding

Another aspect of record keeping for which supervisors were responsible concerned infant feeding. The data recorded from 1951 to 1960 shows a consistently higher number of hospital delivered women chose to artificially feed their babies by the date of discharge. This may have been due to continuity of care or other factors. The interesting issue in this context was that although data was collected on infant feeding it was not fed back to the midwives. Statistics collected were not used for audit by either the supervisor or the MOH, indeed it would be wrong to use much later concepts in the context of this time.

The development of supervision

It is clear from the records and from interviews with supervisors of midwives at this time that they saw their role in terms of protecting mothers and babies and the supervisors in Nottingham carried this out well. There was a large element of inspection in the way they did this. It is equally clear that, through the discussion of critical incidents, the midwife was allowed the opportunity to develop her ability to critically examine her practice and to consider alternative approaches in the safe and facilitative environment of her own home. There is a parallel here between the supervisor's facilitation of the midwife's efforts and the midwife's facilitation of the mother's efforts, each in her own home surroundings. There is no doubt that, during this period, there were supervisors who were seen as dragons rather than facilitators. In Nottingham there is evidence that reflection on practice was facilitated by supervisors and innovations followed. District midwives developed concepts to improve practice and efficiency, such as the introduction of district registers and encouraging each other to take on the postnatal care of women they delivered when 'on call' but who were not their booked clients. Such women often showed a preference for postnatal care from the midwife who delivered their baby. There are many other examples of innovation which arose as a result of supervised practice.

It is important not to use later concepts such as audit and reflective practice in the context of the practice of this time. Such concepts were unknown to these midwives. There was simply no time or opportunity for such enquiry, the workload of these midwives was such that they were constantly running just to stand still. They also worked in the patriarchal culture of their time. Nevertheless, the supervisors enabled the midwives to practice better and by simply addressing the care of individual women their practice anticipated concepts such as reflective practice and critical incident analysis. Woman centred care was the bedrock of their practice. Thus, in many ways, these district midwives were doing what midwifery today seeks to do but does not always accomplish and supervisors were key in facilitating this.

The location of district midwifery services in the heart of the community was central to their effectiveness. Supervisors regularly visited women and midwives in their homes, understanding at first hand the social, economic, racial and political context in which the mothers and babies were living in her area. Responsible directly to the MOH, whose range of responsibility included amongst other things, housing, education and social services, she was best placed to understand the context in which women lived and be in a position to influence. The 1974 National Health Service (Re-organization Act) brought hospital, community and other services into unified Health Authorities. District midwives became employees of the health authorities rather than the local authorities. Regional Health Authorities were nominated as LSAs and supervisors were nominated by the District Health Authorities and approved by the LSAs. As supervision moved away from the MOH and senior district midwives it ceased to be within a public health framework. In 1977 the requirement for a medical supervisor of midwives was abolished. Midwives were therefore supervised by midwives but largely supervised within hospitals and the hierarchical framework of health authorities. From this time supervision had an institutional and professional context, it lacked a context in public health or the lives of childbearing women.

The situation in Nottingham during the years here described is not a paradigm for present day supervision of midwives but it does show that supervision in that era reflected, in the widest sense, the spirit which was intended. Supervision here appeared to be applied correctly both to midwifery practice, with the evidence of support and fostering of reflection on practice, and to women's lives with the close links with basic social issues, such as housing. It can be argued that in recent years the supervision of midwives has not been geared in this wider sense to the needs of women and of midwives but has been primarily concerned with the needs of the organizations which provide midwifery care. Efforts are being made to make supervision sensitive to the needs of midwives but the organizational structures are such that it would be extremely difficult for the supervision of midwives to be grounded in the experience of women's lives. Today Directors of Public Health Medicine act as the guardians of local public health and it seems imperative that in some way the liaison between supervisors of midwives and departments of public health are widened. Whether babies are born in hospital or delivered at home, home is where they will be reared and a clearer understanding of the function of the supervisor could facilitate improvement in maternal and child health.

References

Allison, J. (1996). *Delivered at Home.* London: Chapman and Hall.

City of Nottingham (1962). *Annual Report of the Health Services.* Medical Officer of Health W. Dodd, MD.

HMSO (1959). *Report of the Maternity Services Committee.* London: HMSO.

HMSO (1969). *Local Government Reform Report of the Royal Commission on Local Government in England.* London: HMSO.

HMSO (1970). *Domiciliary Midwifery and Maternity Bed Needs.* London: HMSO.

HMSO (1972). *National Health Service Reorganisation.* London: HMSO.

HMSO Social Services Committee (1980). *Perinatal and Neonatal Mortality.* 2nd Report from the Social Services Committee Session, London: HMSO.

Supervision from the Perspectives of the Statutory Bodies

CHAPTER THREE

The UKCC Perspective: The Statutory Basis for the Supervision of Midwives Today

Jane Winship RM, RGN, MTD DipN (Lond)
has worked as a Professional Officer, Midwifery at the UKCC for the past 10 years and in February 1996 took up a new post in the UKCC which included responsibility for European Affairs for Nursing, Midwifery and Health Visiting. She is President of the European Union Advisory Commitee on the Training of Midwives and a Vice President of the Royal College of Midwives. She is currently completing a MSc degree at the University of Surrey on Change Agent Skills and Strategies.

The privilege of self regulation is the jewel in the crown of a mature profession and we must continue to enable and nurture its development. All professions that enjoy the privilege, through the granting of legal powers to regulate their affairs, need confidence and resolve to stand firm to use that power to develop a high standard of professional practice and integrity for the public good. The use of such legal power in professional practice is not about limiting practice but rather about legitimizing practice and enabling it to grow and develop.

This chapter on the supervision of midwives is written from the perspective of a professional officer for midwifery at the United Central Council for Nursing, Midwifery and Health Visiting (the UKCC) who is a practising midwife by virtue of holding a post for which a midwifery qualification is essential, as is defined in Rule 27 of the Midwives Rules (UKCC, 1993). The role requires the post-holder to provide advice, guidance and interpretation of the midwives legislation, code and standards relating to supervision as well as all other matters relating to midwifery.

Regulation of midwives - 'setting the scene'

The United Kingdom has over 35,000 practising midwives[1] who have had legislation legitimizing their practice since 1902, and even after 94 years the struggle continues to maintain the freedom and autonomy of practice that our legislation affords. Why then did British midwives struggle for so many years to secure their legislation in 1902?

---

[1]. In the text which follows the use of the female gender equally implies the male

Why do midwives all over the world fight for legislation to empower them to regulate their profession? And why are they still endeavouring to secure consumer led practice that is safe, yet not encumbered with unnecessary medical intervention? Canadian midwives are probably the most recent group to seek legislation and the reason stated in a recent article on the struggle for recognition of midwifery in Canada says: 'Unless midwifery is legally recognized, midwives have to be self-employed and practise in the community. With no legislation in place there is no way of controlling standards of care, unless something goes wrong and there is a court case' (Herbert, 1995). What is being said here is that legal recognition for midwives gives freedom to provide the type of safe professional care wanted by women world-wide.

In 1979 we saw the passing of the Nurses, Midwives and Health Visitors Act which was rushed through Parliament just before the resignation of the Labour Government. It was 'An Act to establish a Central Council for Nursing, Midwifery and Health Visiting, and National Boards for the four parts of the United Kingdom; to make new provision with respect to the education, training, regulation and discipline of nurses, midwives and health visitors and the maintenance of a single professional register...'. This Act had not been without its problems for midwives, who had determinedly sought for and succeeded in establishing a special clause to be inserted into the Act enshrining in the legislation the requirement for a statutory midwifery committee that must be consulted on all 'midwifery matters'. This clause addressed their concerns and strengthened the Act for midwives.

The other strength of the Act is that the supervision of midwives continues to be a statutory requirement for the midwifery profession. This is specified in the primary and in the secondary legislation, and it is the UKCC Midwifery Committee that has the responsibility for formulating the Rules to control the practice of midwives, which includes the supervision of midwives. The 1979 Act at Section 4 (4) clearly states that 'The Secretary of State shall not approve rules relating to midwifery practice unless satisfied that they are framed in accordance with recommendations of the Council's (the UKCC) Midwifery Committee'. In legal terms 'shall' is a powerful word and makes it an absolute requirement for the UKCC to satisfy the Secretary of State that the Midwifery Committee is content with all the recommendations for any new or revised rules. Another important strength of this legislation is the requirement at section 4 (1) of the Act for practising midwives to be in the majority on the UKCC Midwifery Committee.

The regulation of midwives and nurses has been a joint process in the United Kingdom since 1983 when the Council took over the regulatory function from the previous nine statutory and training bodies, and this has provided an increased sharing of knowledge and experience between the two professions. However, it was agreed in 1986, in a UKCC report on the future of education, that midwifery is a profession different from, but complementary to nursing. The UKCC Project 2000 Report stated that '... the role of the midwife is... substantially different from the nurse in that a midwife potentially has a greater professional independence as the decision making is of a different order. The midwife is expected to have diagnostic skills relating to both mother and baby that are similar to the obstetrician, and indeed that there is an overlap of skills between the two. Midwives also have a limited responsibility to prescribe certain scheduled drugs and the right of referral to and discharge from hospital within limitations. All these, together with the need for manual dexterity and to develop the confidence required to function in this way, point to a potentially special and different preparation for midwifery' (UKCC, 1986).

Midwifery is also unique in having a system of supervision required in statute. The supervision of midwives is but one aspect of the regulatory process of the profession of midwifery, and must be considered in the context of the whole of the UKCC's regulatory process.

Regulation can imply restriction, but in relation to the professions it has been defined as a system with the necessary formal authority to bring order and consistency to professional affairs. Such order and consistency should at least:

1.   secure minimum standards of education, practice and conduct

2.   enable practice to be relevant and responsive to the changing nature and demands of health needs and care

3.   demonstrably improve standards in the public interest and

4.   call midwives to account if their practice falls below an acceptable standard as designated by the regulatory body (Ralph, 1992).

Primary legislation -the statutory basis for supervision of midwives

The statutory basis for the supervision of midwives can be traced through primary legislation from 1902 to the present primary legislation relating to the UKCC, within the 1979 and 1992 Nurses, Midwives and Health Visitors Acts. These Acts of Parliament have been agreed by the House of Commons and the House of Lords and are Acts that have been secured in the public interest. Such Acts are usually 'enabling' Acts in that they provide a framework from which statutory rules may be derived, otherwise known as secondary or subordinate legislation. Statutory rules do not generally require parliamentary time as they are, when agreed, endorsed by the Secretary of State and laid before the House of Commons for formal and generally automatic approval. Statutory rules can therefore be implemented or amended much more quickly. (Bent, 1992 and Jenkins, 1995 both give useful detail on the processing of statutory law if you need to find out more about this process.)

So, put simply, the 1979 and 1992 Nurses, Midwives and Health Visitors Acts, (which will be referred to in the rest of this chapter as 'the Act', as the 1992 was an amendment to the 1979 Act), lay down the broad framework in law from which the Midwives Rules (the secondary legislation) are drawn up by the UKCC and amended as necessary. The important issue is that these rules are drawn up *by midwives for midwives* and this is the basis of professional self-regulation. Self-regulation is not about limiting practice, but enabling its development and providing a framework for accountable decision making in the interests of public safety.

Relevant sections of the Act

As far as the legal basis for the supervision of midwives is concerned the most important sections of the Act are:

Section 3 - setting up the UKCC Midwifery Committee

This section directs the UKCC to set up two Standing Committees, these being a Midwifery Committee and a Finance Committee.

Section 4 - the UKCC Midwifery Committee

The Midwifery Committee *must* have a majority of practising midwives and *must* be consulted by the UKCC on 'all matters relating to midwifery', and 'the Secretary of State shall not approve rules relating to midwifery practice unless satisfied that they are framed in accordance with recommendations of the Council's Midwifery Committee'.

It is of historical interest here to note that the Nurses, Midwives and Health Visitors Act, 1992, changed the functions of the National Boards, and included the demise of the Standing Midwifery Committees at all four National Boards. However, it is important to note that at the Committee stage of the passage of the Bill that eventually became the 1992 Act, Virginia Bottomley, the then Secretary of State, in response to a question about the Midwifery Committees made the following positive statement:

> 'I reiterate the Governments' commitment to maintaining the unique and separate nature of the midwifery profession. Midwifery shares, and will continue to share, a common regulatory structure with nursing and health visiting, but its 'special' position will continue to be recognized within that structure, as it has been since 1902. At UKCC level, the powers and responsibilities of the Midwifery Committee will remain as they are now' (Hansard, 4 March 1992).

Section 15 - the making of rules regulating the practice of midwives

The important issue here is that the UKCC is mandated to make rules regulating practice and some important examples are given in this section of the Act. It is notable that midwifery is the *only* profession enabled by the Act to make Rules which are standards for regulating *practice*. However, all three of the professions regulated by the Act are required to make rules relating to their education (see Sections 2(2) and 6).

Section 16 - the provision of local supervision of midwifery practice

Section 16(1) designates the bodies who shall be Local Supervising Authorities (LSAs) for midwives in each of the four countries of the United Kingdom:

- In England - Regional Health Authorities
- In Wales - Area Health Authorities
- In Scotland - Health Boards
- In Northern Ireland - Health and Social Services Boards.

It should be noted that the afore mentioned is a direct quote from the Act which will be amended once the 1995 Health Authorities Act is implemented on 1 April 1996. This Act is about further reforming the Health Service in England which will include the abolition of Regional Health Authorities replacing them with Regional Offices of the NHS Executive. New 'Health Authorities' will be formed by the merger of the District Health Authorities with the Family Health Service Authorities. These Health Authorities will take on some of the functional responsibilities of the old Regional Health Authorities. The responsibility for the LSA function will become that of the newly formed Health Authorities. The new Health Authorities Act will lead to the amendments of the Nurses, Midwives and Health Visitors Act, and this will alter the terminology (quoted from section 16(1) above) relating to England and Wales.

Section 16 (2) requires the LSAs to exercise general supervision over *all* midwives practising within their area in accordance with the UKCC Midwives Rules. This means every practising midwife in whatever environment she practices, whether employed or self-employed. Under this section of the Act the LSA is required to report any alleged misconduct on the part of the midwife to the UKCC, and finally it also has power in accordance with the UKCC Midwives Rules to suspend a midwife from practice. This will be discussed in more detail on page 45-46.

Section 16(3) empowers the UKCC to lay down in rules the qualifications necessary for a person to appointed as a supervisor of midwives by the LSA.

Section 16(4) gives the National Boards the responsibility for providing advice and guidance to the LSAs in respect of the exercise of their functions as described in Section 16 of the Act.

Section 16(5) was a new section within the 1992 Act and empowers the UKCC to make rules prescribing the advice and guidance that is given by the National Boards to LSAs. This is in line with the implementation of the 1992 Act giving the UKCC overall responsibility for the supervision of midwives and empowering it to set standards for the entire United Kingdom.

Section 17 - attendance by unqualified persons at childbirth

This is an important section and restricts those who may attend a woman in childbirth. *Sections 17(2) and (3)* state that only a registered midwife or registered medical practitioner, or a student midwife or medical student as part of a statutorily recognized course, may attend a woman in childbirth and it therefore makes the public liable to prosecution if they intentionally undertake this role. Although *Section 17(4)* lays down a fine of not more than £500 to the person who contravenes this part of the Acts, this fine is now linked with a sliding scale introduced by the Criminal Justice Act and can be in excess of £2000.

Male midwives

It should be noted that in relation to the proviso (made at Section 17[2]) for a male registered midwife attending a women in childbirth in a place approved by the Secretary of State, secondary legislation was implemented in 1984 (SI 1983 No1202) which confirmed equality for males and females in the education and practice opportunities for midwives in the United Kingdom.

Secondary legislation - the UKCC's business

As discussed earlier, the primary legislation empowers the UKCC to draw up secondary legislation in the form of rules, in this case the Midwives Rules. This is facilitated through the UKCC Midwifery Committee with its majority membership of practising midwives, and in consultation with the profession. This consultation process is required by the Act in Section (22).

The UKCC constantly reviews its legislation and codes, which set standards to ensure that they are providing an up to date foundation and a framework for development, to enable response to the changing needs of client led care and professional practice. It should be remembered that we have only had 'Midwives Rules' and 'A Midwife's Code of Practice' applicable to the whole United Kingdom since 1986. Since 1986 there have been major revisions to both the education and practice rules and the Code of Practice for midwives, the most recent being 1993 (the Rules) and 1994 (the Code of Practice). It should be appreciated that the Midwives Rules are set in legislation and the Code of Practice, whilst not a legislative document, is UKCC policy, which supports and complements the Rules by setting out in simple terms the standards and other important requirements and information to assist safe practice.

Legislation should be enabling

It is of paramount importance when considering these rules and standards to understand that such legislation is about *enabling practice* and not about limiting practice. It can be seen at a glance if one looks at older editions of rules and codes that there has been a concerted move away from prescriptive rules, to rules that legally define the sphere of practice of the midwife in the interests of the public, so enabling the midwife to use her clinical judgement. It is also interesting to note here that we are still getting a steady trickle of enquiries from midwives who are actually seeking *more* prescriptive direction from the UKCC, and not less. However, the majority of midwives, who are now practising with greater confidence based on sound knowledge and skills, appreciate the flexibility of Rules that are enabling. This is also true for current supervisors of midwives who have been afforded a sound preparation for their role enabling them to be open to the challenge of present day practice alongside the midwives whom they supervise.

The purpose of supervision of midwives

The purpose of supervision of midwives is to protect the public by actively promoting a safe standard of midwifery practice. These standards are agreed by midwives for midwives in the Midwives Rules and Code of Practice. Supervision is not about punitive discipline, nor is it about establishing only one way of providing safe care to the women and babies of this country. It is about quality, about caring and preventing poor practice, and also about seeking excellence with midwives supporting midwives in this process. It is about enabling midwives to practice with competence and confidence in a properly resourced work environment.

There has been a surge of development in the standards relating to the supervision of midwives over the past few years, and the UKCC Midwifery Committee has had a major influence on the way in which the statutory framework and standards have been developed.

Section 16 (5) of the 1992 Act made provision for the further development of specific standards for the supervision of midwives, and this has enabled constructive changes in the existing rules and codes.

The Midwives Rules (1993)

There were important amendments and additions made to the Midwives Rules following the implementation of the Nurse, Midwives and Health Visitors Act 1992 which were of particular relevance to the supervision of midwives. There follows an explanation concerning those changes to the Rules in so much as they are relevant to the supervision of midwives.

RULE 36: NOTIFICATION OF INTENTION TO PRACTICE

Rule 36 enables the supervisor of midwives to identify those midwives whose practice is being supervised, and conversely if used appropriately in a practical sense, equally enables the practising midwife to identify her supervisor of midwives. This rule requires the midwife to 'give notice of her intention to practice to each local supervising authority'. The notice is in a form prescribed by the UKCC, and is now sent directly to every practising midwife on the UKCC register in time for such notification to be made by 31 March each year. It is the midwife's responsibility to comply with this rule, and the notification is returned to the LSA via the supervisor of midwives for the reason stated above. It should be noted that this annual requirement is quite separate and different from the 'Notification of Practice' introduced with the UKCC Post-Registration Education and Practice (PREP) requirements which only identifies an area of practice and relates to three yearly maintenance of registration requirements.

There is nothing in this rule which allows a supervisor of midwives to refuse a notification of intention to practice from a midwife. On occasions enquiries have been received from supervisors about their wish to refuse such a notification of intention to practice because it is believed, for various reasons, that the midwife in question should not be practising. Providing the midwife is a practising midwife as defined in Rule 27 of the Midwives Rules and has demonstrated maintenance of practice as required by the PREP Rules which will be gradually replacing Rule 37 refresher courses, she is eligible to practise as a midwife. If there is a question relating to the standard of a midwife's practice, the notification of intention to practice form is not the mechanism with which such issues should be dealt.

RULE 37: REFRESHER COURSES

Supervisors of midwives have always played an important role in advising midwives about the range of National Board approved programmes and other methods available to fulfil this Rule in relation to both on-going maintenance of practice and return to practice requirements. By 1 April 2000 this Rule will be superseded by the UKCC PREP requirements (UKCC, 1994a). The changes are being introduced gradually according to the dates when current individual requirements are due, and practising midwives are being notified individually of such requirements in relation to their due renewal of registration. However, the important issue here in relation to supervisors of midwives is the different but equally important role they will need to continue to fulfil, and that is the provision of advice and support to midwives relating to their personal review of their competence in order to develop appropriate plans for their own professional development. There is now a wealth of opportunity for midwives to plan their own personal professional development, but assistance will be necessary to make the transition from, what has been for some midwives, a fairly narrow field of opportunity of 'set refresher courses', to a very wide choice governed largely by the innovative ideas of individuals.

RULE 38: SUSPENSION FROM PRACTICE BY A LOCAL SUPERVISING AUTHORITY

There is perhaps more discussion about the use of this rule than any other, which is quite disproportionate to the actual number of occasions that it is required to be implemented. It is because of the misunderstanding surrounding this issue that a lengthy explanation has been included in this chapter.

At the time of writing there are 35,230 practising midwives in the United Kingdom and there are on average 13 - 14 midwives suspended from practice, none of whom are independent midwives. This is contrary to reports in the press and to subjective statements often made from platforms up and down the country, when claims are made, for example, about the high number of independent midwives that are suspended from practice.

Paragraph (2) of this rule states that '... the LSA may suspend from practice until proceedings or investigations have been determined: (a) a midwife against whom it has reported a case for investigation to the Council; (b) a midwife who has been referred to the Professional Conduct Committee of the Council; and (c) a midwife who has been referred to the Health Committee of the Council... '. A Registrar's letter (UKCC, 1994b) emphasizes the discretionary nature of this Rule and says 'If the LSA chooses to suspend a midwife from practice the decision must be able to be justified as being in the interest of the public or the practitioner'. The letter also re-emphasizes the fact that this power cannot be delegated to a supervisor of midwives and that any such decision applies only to the geographical area in which that LSA has jurisdiction. This rule is not there as a threat to practice, it is there to protect the standard of care given to mothers and babies by preventing a midwife who is not able, for a specific reason, to provide a safe standard of care. It is applicable to any practising midwife wherever she is providing care.

Suspension from practice should not be confused with *suspension from duty* which involves an employer suspending an employee from her place of work in relation to an alleged breach of the terms of a contract of employment, and could apply to any health care worker and not only a midwife.

INTERIM SUSPENSION OF REGISTRATION

Interim suspension of registration is not part of the Midwives Rules, but is part of the UKCC Professional Conduct Rules (Statutory Instrument 1993, No.893). It is included here for information and to be considered alongside suspension from practice of midwives.

A new type of 'suspension' was introduced by the UKCC following the 1992 Act when it revised the Professional Conduct Rules, and it can apply to *all* nurses, midwives and health visitors on the UKCC register. This new power is the power of *interim suspension of registration* and can be considered by the Preliminary Proceedings Committee of the UKCC. When a case of alleged misconduct is reported to the UKCC, it is initially considered by the Preliminary Proceedings Committee and if an interim suspension of registration is to be considered, the practitioner is informed that she may be present with a representative, and may present reasons as to why she believes that such a suspension should not be made. If an interim suspension of registration is made, it is applicable across the whole United Kingdom and any such suspension must be reviewed every three months for as long as the suspension is in force.

In the event of a midwife being suspended from practice by an LSA, the midwife would be reported to the UKCC for investigation of the allegations and the case would be considered by the Preliminary Proceedings Committee. If an interim suspension of registration is to be considered, this would give the midwife the right of appearance before the Preliminary Proceedings Committee to give reasons as to why an interim suspension of registration should not be made. In the event of an interim suspension of registration *not* being made, the LSA suspension from practice may require review. There has not been a test of such a situation to date. However, if an interim suspension of registration were made, it would apply throughout the United Kingdom and be subject to a three monthly review which is *not* the case in suspension from practice. The process of interim suspension of registration appears to be a fairer process because of the right of the practitioner to appear and give reasons for the suspension *not* to be imposed and because of the required review process. However, this should be viewed as a possible adjunct to suspension from practice which allows the LSA to take urgent steps to protect the public as was discussed earlier in the section relating to *suspension from practice by a local supervising authority* on page 45.

RULE 40: SPHERE OF PRACTICE

This is probably the most important of the Practice Rules and whilst is remained unchanged in the 1993 Rules, it was further expanded in the 1994 edition of the Midwife's Code of Practice (see pages 48 - 50).

RULE 43: INSPECTION OF PREMISES AND EQUIPMENT

This rule was retained in the 1993 edition of the Midwives Rules, but with changes resulting from the change in the constitution and function of the National Boards and the UKCC, consequent to the 1992 Act. Paragraph (1) of this rule requires a practising midwife to give her supervisor of midwives 'every reasonable facility to inspect her methods of practice, her records, her equipment and such part of her residence as may be used for professional purposes'.

Paragraph (2) was changed and you may be interested to know the reason behind these changes. Paragraph (2) reads: 'A midwife shall use her best endeavours to permit inspection from time to time by a midwifery officer, who shall be a practising midwife, of the Council (the UKCC) or of an authority designated by the Council, of all institutional premises in which she practises other than the private residence of the mother and baby'. The rule previously stated that this function should be carried out by the National Board.

The UKCC Midwifery Committee when discussing and considering the necessary changes to the Midwives Rules was concerned that unless there was specificity, (as laid out in the rule quoted above), a situation could arise where there may not be a practising midwife employed at a National Board to carry out this function. This is not the case at the current time, nor, hopefully will it ever be, and in fact the National Boards continue to carry out this function as the 'authorities designated by the Council' to which all four National Boards have formally agreed. It is in the interest of standards of care for mothers and babies that this function is continued, as it involves visits to those institutions that do not provide education and training for student midwives, but do provide maternity care, but are not the subject of National Board practice visits, as is the case with institutions providing education and training.

RULE 44: SUPERVISORS OF MIDWIVES

This was amended to require that a person to be appointed as a supervisor of midwives must complete a course of instruction *prior* to her appointment, rather than within one year of appointment. This was changed to enable midwives to be properly prepared *before* taking on this key responsibility.

RULE 45: DISCHARGE OF STATUTORY FUNCTIONS BY A LOCAL SUPERVISING AUTHORITY

This rule was added in 1993 to set a standard for the United Kingdom as there were considerable differences in the discharge of LSA functions across the four countries. The UKCC Midwifery Committee believed that to achieve consistency across the United Kingdom, such standards should be set by the professional regulatory body. It was intended that the rule would help to clarify the standards for LSAs and the supervisors of midwives accountable to them.

Rule 45 requires LSAs to determine, implement and publish details of policies at least every two years. Details required are:

1.   the date in the month of March by which notice of intention to practise under Rule 36 must be received by it and;
2.   the name or office of the person to whom the said notice must be sent;
3.   the means by which it will:
     - investigate any prima facie case of misconduct and
     - determine whether to suspend a midwife from practice under Section 16(2)(b) of the Act
4.   a list of the supervisors of midwives whom it has appointed and;
5.   details of how it will provide midwives with continuous access to a supervisor of midwives;
6.   details of how the practice of midwives will be supervised;
7.   all policies which it has formulated affecting the practice of midwives.

The need for the function of the LSA to be carried out by a practising midwife and the need for a standard relating to the number of midwives to be supervised by each supervisor of midwives, was also considered by the Midwifery Committee when it was amending the rules in 1993. It was not possible to put these standards into Rules (Secondary legislation), however they were agreed as UKCC policy in the interest of further developing United Kingdom standards for the supervision of midwives, and these standards have been incorporated in the 1994 Midwife's Code of Practice. It is encouraging to note the positive developments which have ensued from these constructive Council policies.

The Midwife's Code of Practice (1994)

This edition of the Code was considerably revised to take account of new Rules and to make it more 'user friendly' to midwives. It states that the standard of practice in the delivery of midwifery care shall be that which is acceptable in the context of current knowledge and clinical developments, and that in all circumstances the safety and welfare of the mother and baby must be of primary importance. The section relating to responsibility and sphere of practice now includes guidance for the midwife in cases where she believes there is significant risk. This guidance relates in particular to record keeping and communication with the supervisor of midwives in risk situations.

Whilst it is vital for practising midwives to be familiar with the whole of the Code of Practice, some of the important revised and additional paragraphs relating to Rule 40 and the sphere of practice have been quoted below. These paragraphs have been selected because they are of particular relevance to the supervisor of midwives in her support of practising midwives.

PARAGRAPH 13

'Midwives have a defined sphere of practice and you are accountable for that practice. The needs of the mother and baby must be the primary focus of your practice. The mother should be enabled to make decisions about her care based on her needs, having discussed matters fully with you and any other professionals involved with her care'.

PARAGRAPH 14

'You should be appropriately prepared and clinically up to date to ensure you are able effectively to carry out emergency procedures for the mother or baby such as resuscitation'.

PARAGRAPH 17

'When you consider that there could be significant risk in the type of care the mother is requesting, you should discuss her wishes with her, giving detailed information relating to her requests, options for care and any risk factors so that the mother may make a fully informed decision about her care. A detailed record should be made of any such discussion. If the mother rejects your advice, you should seek further advice and discussion with your supervisor of midwives. Such advice and information should be recorded and signed by both you and your supervisor. You must continue to give unbiased care to the best of your ability, seeking peer support as necessary'.

PARAGRAPH 18

'In some instances where risk factors have been identified, or in an emergency, you may require medical assistance for a mother or baby, but the mother or her partner may refuse to have the registered medical practitioner in attendance. If this situation arises you must continue to care for the mother and baby and consult as soon as possible with your supervisor of midwives, making a detailed record of the circumstances and action taken'.

This edition of the Code also included for the first time information about the role of the supervisor of midwives. This may be found in paragraphs 50 and 51 quoted below.

PARAGRAPH 50

'The supervisor of midwives is concerned with safety in practice and care. You and your supervisor of midwives have a mutual responsibility for effective communication between you in order that any problems can be shared and a resolution achieved at the earliest opportunity. A key and important aspect of the supervisory function is that it enables this process'.

PARAGRAPH 51

'Your supervisor of midwives should give you support as a colleague, counsellor and advisor. This should be developed in order to promote a positive working relationship which is conducive to maintaining and improving standards of practice and care'.

Of particular relevance to the supervision of midwives are the inclusion of the two new UKCC policies in paragraphs 45 and 48.

PARAGRAPH 45

'The Council (UKCC) has recommended to LSAs that the LSA function should be discharged by a practising midwife. It is for each LSA to determine its organizational arrangements but the Council considers that this function would be best discharged, and the LSA most appropriately served, by this function being assigned to a practising midwife who is professionally experienced in the supervision of midwives. The Council considers that such a practising midwife should be deployed at LSA level as the designated responsible officer and that the relationship between such a midwife, and the Authority's designated chief nursing/midwifery adviser is of particular importance'.

PARAGRAPH 48

'The Council (UKCC) has recommended to LSAs that for effective supervision to be achieved, each supervisor should supervise no more than 40 practising midwives. The Council understands that there is variation across the United Kingdom in the supervisor-midwife ratio and that it may take some time for some LSAs to reach the recommended ratio. The Council's annual statistical analysis will enable changes to be monitored. This recommendation is designed to allow both effective supervision and adequate support for midwives practising within and outside the National Health Service'.

A number of midwives have asked why the UKCC recommended 40 as being the optimum number for each supervisor to supervise. This figure was reached at that time as being a reasonable number to aim for, given the existing differences in the ratios in the four countries. However, it is hoped that this figure will be lowered over the coming years. As can be seen from the table and graph below taken from the UKCC statistics for the year ending 31 March 1988 to the year ending 31 March 1996, there has been an improvement in these ratios, and particularly in Scotland.

An analysis of the number of midwives per supervisor of midwives

The following statistics show the number of midwives per supervisor in the United Kingdom as a whole from the year ending 31 March 1988 to the year ending 31 March 1996 (Fig 3.1).

Year	England	N. Ireland	Scotland	Wales	UK
1988	46	73	117	46	51
1989	43	77	110	39	47
1990	39	85	107	41	44
1991	39	77	112	42	45
1992	37	88	74	43	41
1993	35	70	80	46	39
1994	33	57	60	41	36
1995	36	68	51	41	38
1996	32	62	39	39	34

Fig. 3.1: Number of midwives per supervisor March 1988-1996
(UKCC, Annual Statistics, 1995b).

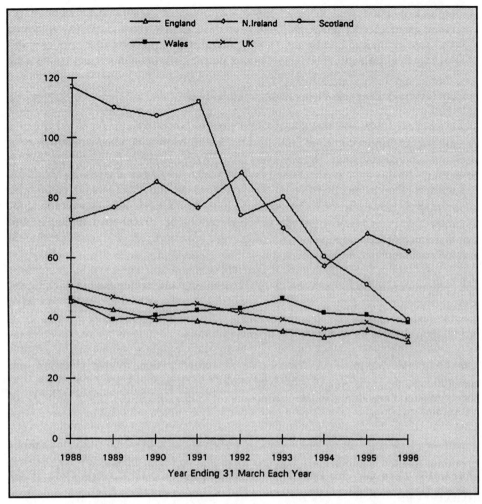

Fig. 3.2: Number of midwives per supervisor in each country compared over a nine year period 31 March 1988 to 31 March 1996 (UKCC Annual Statistics, 1995b)

Background to current developments

In June 1994 the UKCC Midwifery Committee established a Task Group to develop proposals for further standards for the supervision of midwives. It was agreed that it would be appropriate to undertake surveys of LSAs and supervisors of midwives across the United Kingdom. The information obtained would inform the Committee and ensure that decisions made with regard to developing the supervision of midwives in the future would be based on the most recent information.

Conclusions from the LSA survey confirmed the existing understanding of the Midwifery Committee about the situation with regard to LSA activity across the United Kingdom. The response rate was 71 per cent. One third of these LSAs had a practising midwife in post which was encouraging, but indicated a need for the UKCC to continue to publicize its recommendation in this regard to ensure that the number of such LSAs continued to increase. Overall the responses indicated that the supervision of midwives was being given a higher profile than had been the case in the past and it was suggested that the activity undertaken by the UKCC through the promotion of its policies and revised Midwives Rules and Midwife's Code of Practice had been important in achieving this improvement.

Conclusions from the supervisor of midwives survey

Overall the responses confirmed much of the information which had previously only been available anecdotally. The response rate (59 per cent) was rather disappointing, particularly in the light of the dissatisfaction which had been expressed about the supervision of midwives by many of those with whom the UKCC was attempting to communicate. However, the impression given in the response was, as with the LSAs, that the supervision of midwives was being given a higher profile than in the past and that those involved in supervisory activities were anxious to see further development and improvement.

The differences in the preparation of supervisors of midwives offered in each of the four countries of the United Kingdom were demonstrated in the results, and have provided a focus for the developments being considered in relation to consistency in preparation opportunities across the United Kingdom.

Also identified was the need for the use of agreed criteria for the selection and appointment of supervisors of midwives in all LSAs. It was indicated that this would help to ensure consistency in the approach to selection and appointment throughout the United Kingdom.

A working Conference on the supervision of midwives was held by the UKCC in October 1994. This was the first time that all the participants involved in the statutory supervision of midwives had been brought together from the whole of the United Kingdom. These participants included the statutory bodies, LSAs, supervisors of midwives, representatives from consumer associations and others with an involvement and or interest in the supervision of midwives. This undertaking further informed the Midwifery Committee of the needs to be considered in making formative decisions to develop the standards for the supervision of midwives and midwifery practice.

All the information obtained through the working conference on the supervision of midwives and the surveys of the LSAs and the supervisors of midwives was considered and recommendations for the future were agreed by the Midwifery Committee and the UKCC. This resulted in a consultation with the profession on proposed amendments and additions to the Midwives Rules. The consultation took place between June and September 1995 (UKCC, 1995a). The response to the consultation indicated positive support for the proposals.

The resulting recommendations of the Midwifery Committee, as agreed by the UKCC at its meeting in January 1996, set out the *intent of proposed new Rules.* The proposed new rules now have to be put into legal language and go through the usual legislative process within government before they can be circulated to the profession in the form of a revised edition of the Midwives Rules. Until that time the 1993 Midwives Rules will continue to apply.

Proposed amendments and additions to the Midwives Rules

The recommendations of the Midwifery Committee were that further standards should be developed, firstly to further improve the standard of the supervision of midwives and secondly to facilitate consistency in the supervision of midwives in the four countries of the United Kingdom. The *proposals* are as follows:

1. Definition of the supervisor of midwives (Rule 27)

The purpose of this Rule is to provide clear meanings for the expressions which are used throughout the Rules. In the current edition (1993) of the UKCC Midwives Rules the definition of supervisor of midwives is as follows:

> '...means the person appointed by the local supervising authority in accordance with Section 16(3) of the Act'.

A lack of understanding of the role of the supervisor of midwives has been identified as a cause of confusion and therefore of concern by those who participated in the surveys carried out by the UKCC in the past year. It was suggested that an enhancement of the existing definition of the supervisor of midwives may help to clarify the role and function in the future. It is therefore *proposed* that the definition of the supervisor of midwives contained in Rule 27 should be amended to read as follows:

> 'Supervisor of midwives means the person appointed by the LSA in accordance with Section 16(3) of the Act whose responsibilities shall include providing professional support to practising midwives under her supervision in order to establish and improve standards of midwifery practice'.

2. Preparation of supervisors of midwives (Rule 44)

Rule 44 of the Midwives Rules currently requires that a person who is appointed as a supervisor of midwives should have completed a course of preparation in the three years preceding the appointment and that the course should be approved by a National Board. The types of course which are currently undertaken by prospective Supervisors of Midwives in each of the four United Kingdom countries vary in length and form and the UKCC is concerned that there should be consistency in the preparation of supervisors of midwives across the United Kingdom. It is intended that such programmes of preparation should prepare the midwife to assume the responsibilities and accountability for her practice as a midwife when she is appointed to the role of supervisor by the LSA. It is *proposed* that such programmes of preparation should be provided at educational institutes approved by the National Boards.

It is now also considered essential that these programmes of preparation are assessed and accredited, with an appropriate level of academic assessment as an integral part of the programme of preparation, and it is *suggested* that the programmes should be accredited within Higher Education at no less than academic Level 2 in England with the appropriate equivalent accreditation in Scotland, Wales and Northern Ireland.

The UKCC also *proposed* the development of a set of broad learning outcomes to be included in legislation as a method of ensuring a consistent approach to the preparation of supervisors of midwives in the future. It is *proposed* that on completion of a programme of preparation the prospective supervisor of midwives will demonstrate:

1. an understanding of the way in which supervision of midwives enhances standards of care;

2. an understanding of the application of legislation relevant to the supervision of midwives;

3. the ability to provide professional support to practising midwives relevant to maintaining and promoting standards of care;

4. the ability to encourage midwives to use their experience in practice to enhance their professional development;

5. an understanding of accountability and professional responsibility as a supervisor of midwives.

Rule 44, paragraph (2), currently requires supervisors of midwives to undertake 'further instruction' every five years. In support of supervisors of midwives' professional development, it is *recommended* that such professional updating be undertaken every three years rather than every five years, to introduce consistency in all requirements for professional updating.

Finally, in relation to Rule 44, it is *recommended* that the Rule be amended to require a record to be kept on the UKCC register of:

1. completion of a National Board approved programme of preparation as a supervisor of midwives and

2. completion of subsequent development programmes during the periods of time prescribed in the rule.

There is currently no mechanism for entering a record of either programmes of preparation or updating for supervisors of midwives on the UKCC register. This new rule would give professional and academic credence to these programmes in the same way as other approved programmes that are already recorded on the UKCC register.

3. Selection and appointment of supervisors of midwives

It was considered that consistency in the approach to the selection and appointment of supervisors of midwives was essential if United Kingdom standards were to be established and improved. In order to achieve such consistency the UKCC believed that it would be appropriate to develop standards which would require the National Boards to identify appropriate mechanisms for the selection and appointment of supervisors of midwives. To this end the UKCC *proposed* the identification of standards which would enable consistency and good practice in relation to selection and appointment and it is envisaged that they would include the following:

1. self nomination for selection would be appropriate, and ideally, eligible nominees would be supported by those practitioners they might supervise;

2. appointment should be made by a selection panel consisting of some of the following:
   - representative of the LSA
   - experienced supervisor of midwives
   - midwifery manager
   - practising midwife
   - midwifery educationalist

3. a mechanism should be made explicit and recommended for use in reviewing the appointment of supervisors of midwives in cases where the supervisor of midwives has failed to carry out her role appropriately (UKCC, 1995a and 1996).

Future developments

It is recognized that there is still some lack of understanding about the purpose of the supervision of midwives and the role of the supervisor of midwives. This is apparent, both in the profession and among those who are involved in the wider healthcare arena.

When the UKCC has amended and added the agreed rule changes, it intends to publish and distribute widely a document which clearly describes the purpose and function of the supervision of midwives, the role of the supervisor of midwives and the role of the LSA. It is hoped that this will help to reduce the problems which are caused by lack of knowledge or misunderstanding. It is acknowledged that difficulties continue to be experienced by those midwives who practise in more than one LSA, because of the processes for notification of intention to practise and the numbers of supervisors of midwives involved for these midwives. It is intended that this new document will also provide specific help and guidance for this group of midwives.

The need to audit the results of supervision of midwives has been identified and the lack of such audit gives cause for concern. The UKCC Midwifery Committee intends to develop and disseminate principles for use in audit of the supervision of midwives and in the future the results of such audit will then be used to assist in redefining the UKCC standards for the supervision of midwives.

Finally, let us remember as we move forward in times of great change that the supervision of midwives '... enables midwives to identify, through open and honest dialogue, their continuing professional and educational needs. This ultimately enhances the practice and profession of midwifery' (Davis, 1994). The supervision of midwives is not a static scenario, but is dynamic, questioning and moving forwards at all times. It is known and acknowledged that standards for the supervision of midwives vary, but in the main there has been publicity about the negative rather than the positive developments, and it is because of this variation that the UKCC is working towards creating consistent United Kingdom standards. It should also be remembered that we have had Midwives Rules and a Midwife's Code of Practice applying to the whole United Kingdom only since 1986. These have been regularly revised following consultation with the profession, in response to the changing needs and nature of both maternity care and the midwifery profession. In this light it is hoped that 'LSAs and supervisors of midwives will build on the present excellent mechanism to develop and strengthen supervision of midwives as part of its initiative to promote and monitor good practice' (Roch, 1990).

References

Association of Radical Midwives (1995). *Super-Vision, Consensus Conference Proceedings*. Hale: Books for Midwives Press.

Bent, E.A. (1992). *Module 1, Preparation of Supervisors of Midwives: An Open Learning Programme*. London: English National Board.

Davis, K.C. (1994). 'Is statutory supervision central to our professional identity?' *British Journal of Midwifery*, July, Vol 2. No.7 pp.304-305.

Dimond, B.C. (1994). *The Legal Aspects of Midwifery*. Hale: Books for Midwives Press.

Herbert, P. (1995). 'Midwifery in Canada: the struggle for recognition' *Modern Midwife*, February, pp.11-14.

House of Commons (1979). *Nurses, Midwives and Health Visitors Act*. London: HMSO.

House of Commons (1992). *Nurses, Midwives and Health Visitors Act*. London: HMSO.

House of Commons (1992). *Hansard, 4 March*. London: HMSO.

House of Commons (1995). *Health Authorities Act*. London: HMSO.

Jenkins, R. (1995). *The Law and the Midwife*. Oxford: Blackwell Science Ltd.

Ralph, C.J. (1992). 'Standards and accountability' *Keynote Address at Commonwealth Meeting of Chief Nursing Officers and Professional Associations*.

Roch, S.E.G. (1990). 'Midwifery: past, future, perfect?' *Midwife Health Visitor & Community Nurse*, April, Vol. 26, No. 4, pp.110-112.

Statutory Instrument No. 1202 (1993). *Sex Discrimination Act 1975 (amendment of Section 20)*. Order 1983.

Steene, J. (1995). 'A prominent role for local supervising authorities' *British Journal of Midwifery*, June, Vol 3, No. 6, pp.306-307.

UKCC (1986). *Project 2000: A New Preparation for Practice*. London: UKCC p.50.

UKCC (1993). *Midwives Rules*. London: UKCC.

UKCC (1994). *Annual Report 1993-1994*. London: UKCC.

UKCC (1994a). *The Future of Professional Practice - The Council's Standards for Education and Practice Following Registration*. London: UKCC.

UKCC (1994b). Registrar's Letter 8/1994 replacing circular PC/89/02 November 1989.

UKCC (1994c). *A Midwife's Code of Practice*. London: UKCC.

UKCC (1995a). Registrar's Letter 20/1995.

UKCC (1995b). *Annual Statistics for the Year 1 April 1994 to 31 March 1995*. London: UKCC.

UKCC (1996). *Proposed Changes to the Midwives Rules* Paper CC/96/02.

Winship, E.J. (1993). 'The freedom of legislation...where midwives dare..?' in *International Confederation of Midwives 23rd International Congress Proceedings* Vancouver.

Winship, E.J. (1993). 'Regulation: The international midwifery picture' in *Proceedings of the First International Standing Conference on the Regulation of Nursing and Midwifery.* London: UKCC.

CHAPTER FOUR

The ENB Perspective: Preparation of Supervisors of Midwives for their Role

Meryl Thomas SRN, SCM, ADM, MTD, Dip Ed Man, MA
is Director - Midwifery Education and Practice - at the English National Board for Nursing, Midwifery and Health Visiting, with particular responsibility for collaborating on midwifery issues. As Director, she leads the work to achieve the strategic objectives of the Board relating to midwifery education, supervision of midwives and midwifery practice. Previously as a registered nurse and midwife, she held various nursing and midwifery posts, as well as working within midwifery education.

Glynnis Mayes BSc, RGN, RM, RHV, NDN
is Assistant Director for Midwifery Supervision and Practice at the English National Board for Nursing, Midwifery and Health Visiting. Within this, she has been involved in developing and implementing the Board's strategy for the preparation of supervisors of midwives in England. Prior to joining the ENB she was a supervisor of midwives and managed services for women and children for a number of years.

The background to preparation of supervisors of midwives

The 1974 reorganization of the National Health Service established the Regional Health Authorities as Local Supervising Authorities (LSAs). The new Health Authorities had responsibility for both hospital and community maternity services and this opened up new opportunities in the development of supervision of midwives. Midwives within maternity units became designated supervisors of midwives within an integrated midwifery service in partnership with their midwife colleagues already functioning as supervisors of midwives within the community midwifery setting.

By 1977 all supervisors of midwives were required to be practising midwives. Medical supervisors, established through the 1902 Midwives Act, were abolished. The Statutory Instrument (SI 1977 No.1850) which brought this about, also established the requirement for all supervisors of midwives to undergo preparation for that role following designation by the LSA.

In 1978, the Central Midwives Board (CMB) the statutory body at that time, introduced the first induction courses for supervisors of midwives. This was a two-day induction to be undertaken within the first year following appointment by the LSA. 1983 saw the establishment of the United Kingdom Central Council for Nursing, Midwifery and Health Visiting (UKCC) and four National Boards of England, Wales, Scotland and Northern Ireland.

The 1979 Nurses, Midwives and Health Visitors Act had transferred the regulation of midwifery education and practice to the UKCC. The 1992 amendments to the Act also gave the UKCC responsibility for setting standards for supervision of midwives. The UKCC produces Midwives Rules which regulate the education of midwives, the supervision of midwives and midwifery practice. The UKCC sets standards for the qualifications, appointment and preparation of supervisors of midwives and the duties of the LSAs. The four National Boards are responsible for ensuring these standards are met and for giving advice and guidance to LSAs in respect of their function.

The National Boards have the responsibility for providing courses of preparation for supervisors of midwives. The UKCC Midwives Rules (November, 1993) require the course of preparation to be undertaken by the midwife prior to appointment as a supervisor of midwives by the LSA.

In the recent UKCC consultation on proposed changes to the Midwives Rules, the Council intends to strengthen the standards relating to preparation of supervisors of midwives further. This will be achieved first through establishing a set of learning outcomes for the preparation, and secondly, by requiring the National Boards to advise LSAs on standards for selection and appointment of supervisors of midwives.

In addition, a record will be established on Council's Register of successful completion of the supervisors of midwives' preparatory programme and subsequent updating programmes (Steene, 1995).

The programme of Preparation for Supervisors of Midwives introduced by the English National Board (ENB, 1992) requires diploma level study. Since its publication the open learning programme has been utilized in differing ways for preparation of supervisors of midwives by each of the National Boards across the United Kingdom. The programme is being revised by 1996 to take account of the changes in legislation, culture and approach within the maternity services and the wider NHS. In addition, the new UKCC standards relating to supervision of midwives and midwifery practice and its PREP (1995) requirements will be incorporated.

Factors influencing developments 1990-1995

There have been many factors which have influenced the development, by the National Board in England, of the new approach to preparing supervisors of midwives for this most important responsibility. In the 1980s there were several notable incidents of midwives reported to the UKCC for alleged misconduct. Emerging from these cases and the debates and issues surrounding them (Ischerwood, 1988) was a recognition of a lack of common understanding of the responsibilities and limits of authority of supervisors of midwives within the profession. The regional nurses, responsible for the LSA functions, began to question the effectiveness and continued relevance of supervision of midwives. It was certainly the case that the standards, frameworks and execution of the LSA and supervisory responsibilities differed greatly across the country with no common agreement on approaches to supervision across LSAs and even less so across maternity services.

Alongside this growing dissatisfaction with supervision of midwives, there was increasing focus on developing standards of care and measuring outcomes. In developing midwifery services and midwifery curricula, there was an increasing recognition of the need for evidence based practice and a consequent support for midwifery related research. By the late 1980s midwives and women were beginning to react against the medical model of care for women in pregnancy and childbirth which had gained momentum in the previous two decades.

Through its statutory responsibility for providing advice and guidance to LSAs and for undertaking visits to all maternity services, the ENB became acutely aware of these issues. The ENB wished to empower supervisors of midwives to acquire the skills to influence the development of midwives who could give high quality, appropriate midwifery care. Central to this, was a need to strengthen and maintain effective relationships with LSAs and for the ENB to undertake with them a nationwide review of the systems for supervision of midwives and midwifery practice.

The then Professional Advisor (Midwifery) at the ENB, Miss Ann Stewart, undertook a review of the systems for supervision in 1990. There were a number of recommendations arising from the review. One of these was the need to develop a structured educational programme for the preparation of supervisors of midwives.

The development of the Open Learning Programme

It was decided that, in devolving the preparation of supervisors of midwives, open learning would be an appropriate approach and the ENB commissioned the development of an open learning programme for the future preparation. Through the involvement of the ENB midwifery officers, Midwifery Committee members, six expert authors and critical readers, an open learning programme emerged in four modules. Following developmental testing the open learning programme, Preparation of Supervisors of Midwives (ENB, 1992) was launched by the ENB in September of that year.

The philosophy of the pack was underpinned by the contemporary approaches to education as a process with the learner being the pivotal focus. For the first time a common foundation and interpretation of supervision of midwives was promoted as a model for good practice which could be applied throughout the country. The programme was received positively by the profession and has become a widely used source of reference, and elements have been incorporated in other midwifery education programmes.

Operational strategy for programmes on preparation

The ENB agreed with the 14 LSAs the formation of five consortia, each with a designated study centre (Midwife Education Department), to operate the programme. The funding for the programmes was shared between the ENB which provided the open learning materials and the LSAs who funded the operational costs.

The programme requires each midwife to have an allocated supervisor of midwives as a mentor for the duration of the programme. During the first year the ENB provided 180 mentors with the necessary preparation. In the second year this responsibility was transferred to the LSAs in liaison with the designated study centres.

As part of its drive to improve the standards and effectiveness of the systems of supervision the ENB took a bold decision. It required that each midwife nominated by an LSA must successfully complete the programme before embarking on the role as an appointed supervisor of midwives. This was later adopted by the UKCC within the Midwives Rules issued in November 1993.

A number of other elements were also introduced into the programme requirements.

1.   The programme was to include a minimum of two study days at the study centre for peer discussion and sharing of experiences.
2.   The midwife would attend an ENB study day at the end of the programme.
3.   The programme would be operated at the level of diploma in higher education.
4.   There should be opportunity to secure academic credits.

A further element which aroused considerable discussion and some anxiety but which was eventually agreed was the requirement that successful completion would be subject to assessment.

The ENB visited each of the five study centres to approve them to operate the programme. The first programme commenced in June 1993 and the remainder commenced in the Autumn. It was interesting to note the individual characteristics of the programmes as interpreted by each study centre in conjunction with the respective LSA consortium. Some programmes have a pre-programme introductory day and one requires completion of a study skills programme and assertiveness training prior to the commencement of the open learning programme. The majority of the programmes include more than the minimum of two study days. The assessment strategies are individually designed for each programme but the use of a reflective diary and a seminar presentation by participants is a requirement of all programmes. Only one programme has not sought academic accreditation and only one does not require a compulsory written assignment.

The effectiveness of the programme and emerging issues

The programmes have all been viewed positively by the midwives who have completed the study and become supervisors of midwives despite the difficulties which some have encountered. The new approach to the preparation for the role and the widespread use of the open learning pack in particular, have had a major impact on the quality of supervision. The LSAs and existing supervisors have noted and welcomed the improvement in knowledge base and resulting confidence in supervisory activities that have resulted from the introduction of the new preparation. The report of an audit of supervision undertaken by North West Regional Health Authority (Duerden, 1995) reported that 100 per cent of supervisors who had completed the open learning programme felt adequately prepared for the role compared to only eight per cent who had undertaken the previous induction days.

The enthusiasm of the supervisors prepared through the open learning programme has been evident and they are generally reported to have a clearer understanding of their role, cultivating a proactive and positive approach to supervision. This has led to the establishment of effective local systems for supervision, which have been found through practice visits to maternity units by ENB officers to be well utilized by the midwives. As a result, the profile of supervision and the recognition of its value has been raised at the majority of maternity services during the last three years (ENB, 1995).

The introduction of such a major change which involved a shared responsibility between the ENB, the LSAs and the designated study centres was complex. While there were inevitable teething problems, these have been dealt with effectively and the programmes are now operating relatively smoothly.

Commitment to the programme

Open learning offers the flexibility to meet the individual needs and commitments of course members and this has been appreciated by the new supervisors. At the time of undertaking the programme many were settling into new posts, finding themselves in a new management role in the service, in addition to becoming a new supervisor of midwives. For others, the programme has coincided with organization review and restructuring, resulting either in the possibility of redundancy or of losing experienced supervisor colleagues as mentors.

The commitment required of the mentors and tutor counsellors in providing support and guidance for midwives undertaking the programme is extremely demanding on top of their existing workloads. Many gave this support in their own time and this proved to be a lifeline for the nominated supervisors.

The sharing of ideas with fellow programme members, mentors and tutors on study days is an important element of the open learning approach, enabling them to clarify and consolidate the knowledge gained through studying the open learning pack.

In some cases the distance of course members from the study centres has created difficulties both for travelling on the study days and for seeking help in between. Some of the midwives undertaking the programme have experienced difficulties in accessing mentors and tutors. In some cases this has been associated with the distance between the learner supervisor and the mentor supervisor's workplace or the heavy workload pressures experienced by the mentor. This has led to ingenious arrangements to make best use of the time with the mentor and where help has been sought from the tutor-counsellor, this has often been given over the telephone or by post.

There have been a small number of instances of conflicting advice from mentors, tutors and the open learning modules and this has been a cause of major difficulty. Supervision of midwives has long been fraught with differences in interpretation and approach and can be particularly problematic in the preparation of new supervisors. The nominated supervisor feels vulnerable and uncertain in this situation and it detracts from effective study of the programme. The preparation of the tutors and the mentors is therefore crucial to the success of the programme and to the benefits of the open learning approach being realized.

The amount of study leave granted to individuals undertaking the programme has been quite variable. Some have received generous support which they have appreciated. Others have felt the demands of open learning have not been recognized by employers or colleagues resulting in far less time being awarded for study than would have been for a taught course.

The assessment strategies have been a cause of controversy for a variety of reasons. Supervisors soon realize that there is a range of approaches to assessment across the five study centres. Programmes leading to award of academic credit have to meet the requirements of the higher education institution which inevitably includes a written assignment. Where a written assignment is optional there is greater opportunity to pursue the wider aspects of supervision more thoroughly whilst assessing knowledge and practice through other approaches such as seminar presentation. Some nominated supervisors have found the written assignment a valuable learning experience and feel a sense of achievement when successful. For others, it dominated the whole programme and made for a less rich experience.

Success rates and outcomes

Assessment was a new element in the preparation of supervisors of midwives and initially, some study centres experienced a worrying failure rate which was daunting for programme members. In overcoming the difficulty, attention was given to developing more stringent selection criteria including a requirement for individuals to have undertaken recent study. The study centres have also worked hard on clarifying for programme members what was required of them and the criteria used for awarding marks. In addition, study skills packages have been made available to prospective programme members.

1.   By December 1995, 480 midwives had completed the programme and these new supervisors make up a substantial proportion of the total number. This figure includes new supervisors from Wales who have undertaken the programme in England. The newly qualified supervisors represent a diverse range of midwifery practice compared with the former position where the majority of supervisors were also midwifery managers. The profile of the new supervisors in England is shown in Figure 4.1. (see overleaf).

NEWLY QUALIFIED SUPERVISORS (1995)	
54%	Clinical practice
34%	Midwifery management
5%	Other
3.5%	Midwife teachers
3%	Not known

Fig. 4.1: Profile of new supervisors in England (ENB)

The demand for places has risen steadily and each of the five study centres have been granted an increase in the numbers for each intake. The number of midwives completing the programme each year is shown in Figure 4.2.

COMPLETION OF SUPERVISOR'S PROGRAMME	
1993	78
1994	132
1995	270

Fig. 4.2: Numbers of midwives completing the programmes(ENB)

This increase has arisen in many cases from the refiguring of organizational structures within the maternity services, but in others, it is associated with new approaches to developing supervision of midwives. Some units are following a strategy of reducing the ratio of midwives to 10–15 to each supervisor, to allow for closer working relationships which could accommodate elements of clinical supervision.

Preparing for the future

In enabling the profession to prepare for the future through appropriate preparation of supervisors of midwives, the experiences described previously in this chapter will be invaluable. The guiding principles for the future preparation arise from the four major changes currently impacting on midwives and midwifery practice. First, the changes in the NHS structure through the Health Authorities Act (1995). Secondly, the changes in organizational structures and management culture within NHS Trusts. Thirdly, 'Changing Childbirth' (DOH, 1993) and the Government's indicators of success offer opportunities to strengthen the midwives' role (Mayes, 1995). Supervision is a built-in quality assurance system which should be an enabling and supportive framework for midwives as individuals, or in groups, to ensure that they capitalize on the opportunities that developing woman-centred care offers the profession. Lastly, but also the change which may offer the greatest opportunity for further developing the preparation of supervisors of midwives, are the standards for supervision of midwives which the UKCC will be publishing within the new midwives Rules in 1996. It is worth exploring these changes more widely to consider the impact these may have upon the supervision of midwives and midwifery practice and, as a result, on the way in which supervisors should be prepared for their role.

The changes in the National Health Service

In April 1996, responsibility for the LSA functions passed from the Regional Offices to the new Health Authorities. We are fortunate to have retained in statute the LSA function. The benefits of statutory supervision of midwives will need to be evident to the new LSAs. This will be achieved through supervisors of midwives who can contribute to the contracting processes and to achieving standards of midwifery service which meet the contracts. Supervision can play a major role in the formulation of policies, in quality audit and risk management and in providing professional leadership within the maternity services. In order to be effective in these areas, supervisors must increasingly develop political awareness, use firm evidence as the basis for their decisions and be articulate and skilled in putting forward their views at senior management level.

Flattening of the organizational structures has reduced the numbers of midwife managers and, in many instances, lowered the grade of the Head of Midwifery. This has created a rapid turnover in supervisors and many experienced supervisors have been lost from the profession. It is important that the preparation of the new supervisors equips them with the knowledge and skills they need to carry out their supervisory role in positively contributing to developing midwifery practice and the total service to support the interests of mothers and their families.

Supervisors are now selected from a wide range of positions within the organization. There are some supervisors in 'E' and 'F' grade posts, an increasing number are in 'G' grade posts, the remaining majority being at 'H' grade or senior management grades.

There have been a variety of reactions to this situation and there are a number of implications to be considered. It could be viewed as a positive move to have supervisors within the 'E' and 'F' grades demonstrating that supervision is quite separate from management and giving more credibility to practitioners. Conversely, it would not be advisable for supervision to be operating solely at that level if it is to impact upon policy development and quality measurement at Trust level. While a supervisor who is a peer will have a day-to-day working knowledge of a midwife's standards and approach to practice she may not have the experience, confidence or the authority to plan and execute appropriate measures to deal with problems. Where supervisors of midwives are at 'E' or 'F' grade it should be within a service where there are also supervisors at senior manager level. In this way, there are benefits at clinical level and at policy making level and opportunity for supervisors to be developed in their role by those more experienced who can offer effective role models.

The disempowerment experienced within midwifery services is an increasing problem that supervisors face. This has been evident through practice visits and discussions with managers seeking advice from the Board's officers. The disempowerment appears to relate to a number of factors. Strategic planning and determination of policies are often now in the hands of the Trust nurse. Since the establishment of Trusts there has been an ongoing decline in the number of senior posts within the maternity services. This in itself, has seen the loss of experienced managers with the vision gained through such experience. The flattening of structures occurring within the maternity services with implications for staffing levels and skill mix all mitigate against effective professional leadership. It is important that, through the shift of the LSA function to purchaser level, the midwife advisor to the LSA takes opportunity to influence the contracting processes.

It offers opportunity for the contract specifications to strengthen the role of supervision and to enable the supervisor, in a lead management position within the maternity service, to have access to the Trust Board. The major role that supervision can and should play in providing professional leadership, supporting excellence in practice and in enabling quality services which meet consumer needs, must be promoted at LSA and Trust Board level. The challenge for the preparatory programme and for the current and future updating programmes is that they enable the supervisor of midwives to identify the ways in which she can promote the role and enable its value to be evidenced at clinical, Trust Board and purchasing authority level.

The impact of 'Changing Childbirth'

Supervisors of midwives can be the drivers of change and a valuable resource for midwives in enabling them to meet the challenges of 'Changing Childbirth' (Department of Health, 1993). The development of woman-centred care is government policy and offers midwives the opportunity to develop practice and strengthen their role. With the development of the role comes increased autonomy and therefore personal accountability. For many midwives who for years have worked within a medical model of care this can be a daunting and even threatening challenge. Many are reluctantly being driven by the changes instead of being drivers of the change. The last two decades saw the diminution of the midwives' role, the medical model and increased interventionist approaches have stifled rather than developed professional expertise (Mayes, 1995). If there is to be a new approach to offering maternity services then operational frameworks, policies relating to practice and responsibilities of individuals within the service must change.

Supervision of midwives should be the key to unlocking the potential of midwives to achieve the changes envisaged by 'Changing Childbirth' and to replace old systems with new frameworks for care. These frameworks should facilitate flexibility and responsiveness to womens' needs and choices. The supervisor of midwives is the ideal person to ensure that in achieving woman-centred services, due attention is given to policies and protocols required within the standards of a Trust. Support of the Trust Board is important for the success of any change process. The supervisor has an important role in assuring the Trust that the policies being implemented to achieve the targets set by the Government for woman-centred services do not increase the risk of litigation. In those instances where women choose styles of care which may not fit with existing Trust policies, the supervisor of midwives will ensure that any risks will be minimized through the provision of appropriate care. Supervision makes an important contribution to risk management, quality and audit strategies as well as multi-professional development of protocols and guidelines for practice. The value of supervision, when undertaken well, ensures that midwives' practice is based on contemporary evidence and any perceived deficiencies are identified and appropriate corrective measures taken. The supervisor of midwives ensures that the midwives she supervises are clear and confident about the parameters of their role and are competent to fulfil all aspects of the role as sanctioned within a Trust.

This is one of the most difficult aspects to be dealt with in preparing as a supervisor of midwives. Supervision must no longer be viewed as restrictive. In addition, it is important that on completion of the programme the new supervisor has clearly grasped the difference between, but related aspects of, the role of supervisor of midwives and manager of service. Supervisors have been perceived as restrictive and controlling by many midwives (Flint, 1993). An over-emphasis on directing midwives in their practice with too little emphasis on supporting the midwife in practising autonomously, as supported by the legislation, has led to this perception.

The programme of preparation and the role modelling by the supervisors as mentors during the programme should enable the development of supervisors who have a clear understanding of the empowerment offered by the current legislation. In addition, they can articulate that understanding in contributing to the review and development of both frameworks for supervision at LSA and local level and also of policies and frameworks for the development of woman-centred maternity services. The programme of preparation must give the supervisor some confidence in her ability to support midwives in developing their accountability and in dealing effectively with dilemmas relating to practice issues. The supervisor has an important role in supporting the development of new approaches to care and at the same time she must ensure that clinical outcomes are satisfactory and that there has been adequate assessment of potential risks. It is this balance between the professional practice issues central to the supervisory role and the employment, cost effective and expediency focus of the management role that successful supervisors have been able to achieve. Where this balance has been achieved supervision has been valued by the midwives practising within that service and the benefits of the supervisors' advice have been felt at Trust Board level.

The UKCC midwives rules – proposals for change

The UKCC have consulted the profession on the proposed changes to the Midwives Rules. The definition of the supervisor of midwives is to be strengthened. This will give greater clarity for those at LSA and Trust level of what the purpose of the role is. At a time when nurses are exploring systems of clinical supervision, it is important that the statutory aspects of the role and the wider remit of supervision of midwives are articulated within the secondary legislation.

There will be stated outcomes for the supervisors preparatory programme. These will be consistent with the outcomes required by the current ENB preparatory programme but will need to be met across all four member countries of the United Kingdom. There will be a requirement that these outcomes have formal academic assessment and that the programmes are operated within higher education. There will be a need for the National Boards to issue guidance to those in higher education on the requirement for close liaison with the LSAs in relation to programme development and organization. In addition, education purchasing consortia must consult with the LSA responsible officer in relation to purchasing needs and the award of contracts to higher education for the programme.

The UKCC will require the National Boards to give advice and guidance to LSAs on selection and appointment procedures relating to supervisors of midwives. Many of the LSAs in England have already developed effective selection and appointment procedures over the last few years. One of the issues that is now a point of discussion is how the LSAs can introduce a strategy for de-selecting supervisors whose performance is unsatisfactory. The selection and appointment criteria are most important in the light of the demands which are placed upon individuals when they take on the role of supervisor of midwives. A number of approaches are being introduced with some LSAs supporting pilot schemes for peer nomination or self-selection which are then followed up by selection interview at LSA level. These approaches, and the more traditional model of local nomination by existing supervisors to LSAs, will need to be monitored so that the National Boards can ensure that the quality of supervision is maintained and improved by having the most effective and appropriate selection procedures.

The UKCC intend that the completion of the programme will be recorded on the UKCC Register and in addition that the supervisors' update days, which will increase from three to five, will also be recorded. While there will be local flexibility for developing and operating both the preparatory programme and the updating programme, it will for the first time be possible to have a country wide database for information on the numbers of supervisors being prepared and updated through these programmes. It is anticipated that the UKCC will require that these programmes are to be undertaken separate from, and in addition to, the statutory updating required for all midwives within the PREP standards.

The plans for the future of the programme of preparation for supervisors of midwives

A working group has already been formed at the ENB to review and develop the open learning programme which was launched in 1992. The changes to the modules will be wide-ranging and be based on the advice of expert supervisors, LSA responsible officers, clinically based midwives and midwife teachers working with the ENB and the contracted development team. The programme must be developed to incorporate the requirements to equip supervisors of midwives to lead the development of practice. They must be enabled to do this in the context of the current structures and influences in maternity services and the contemporary values of midwives and women using the midwifery services. The programme must enable the supervisor to have a vision about how to contribute to meeting national and local targets, in addition to identifying how supervision can achieve a high profile for midwives within a maternity service and foster effective interprofessional relationships. The supervisor, as a champion of midwives, must develop an approach which is supportive of midwives as competent, autonomous practitioners accountable and responsible for their practice.

The supervisor should have a clear idea of how the tools and empowerment of the role can be used effectively to enable practice to develop. In particular, supervision must be effective in meeting consumer needs and not ignoring the wider issues of multicultural needs and such aspects as incorporating complementary therapies into midwifery practice. It is not an easy role to accomplish, and every supervisor of midwives needs the support of the local network of supervisors in order to develop the local systems and standards so that the LSA standards are achieved.

The supervisor's approach to the support and guidance of midwives working outside the NHS structures will be an important aspect of the preparatory programme. It is accepted that a supervisor is a guardian of practice and issues of safety for the mothers and their babies will always be a prime responsibility. There is a danger in exercising their role with those who fall outside the management structures of the maternity service, that the supervisor uses restrictive and fault finding approaches. The preparatory programme should enable the supervisor to define clearly the responsibility towards the midwife carrying full accountability for the women in her care. The role of the supervisor in this situation should focus on helping the midwife to feel confident about her practice and able to recognize when she should seek help and guidance. Ultimately, the supervisors' role is to ensure that the care of women and their babies is appropriate and within the legitimate boundaries of the role of the midwife.

In producing an updated version of the open learning programme all the issues discussed in this chapter will have a bearing on the content. There will also need to be new guidance for the LSAs and for the study centres operating the programmes. It is likely that a few more centres will offer the programme and this will be welcomed by those LSAs who have been geographically distanced from the current study centres.

The funding issues will form part of the discussions between the National Boards and the new LSAs and the academic level of the programme and the related assessment will need to be effectively negotiated and incorporated when the updated programme is introduced in 1996.

Conclusion

The effectiveness of supervision and its future success and acceptability to both midwives and the health service is dependent on the expertise with which it is carried out. In addition, the value of supervision will only be recognized through the benefit it brings to the development of the midwifery service for improved outcomes.

To have long-term survival the role must be seen to be effective and therefore valued by Health Service purchasers and providers in achieving targets. Midwives who can access and receive the support they require to practice appropriately within or outside the Health Service will also value supervision. Most powerful of all voices are those of the consumers who wish to experience a positive and supportive approach to enabling their needs to be met.

The appropriate midwives must therefore be selected for undertaking this crucial role. The programme of preparation must enable them to acquire the necessary expertise to fulfil all the demands of the supervisors role. The ongoing development of the programme of preparation seeks to address the deficiencies recognized in supervision in the past, and to achieve the professional support and leadership required for the future.

The future of the profession depends greatly on effective leadership and supervisors are pivotal to this need. The future of supervision will be determined by the future needs of midwives and the women for whom the service exists. The educational programme for preparation must reflect the vision of enabling the highest standards of practice to be achieved.

References

Department of Health (1979). *Nurses, Midwives and Health Visitors Act.* Ch.16. London: HMSO.

Department of Health (1993). *Changing Childbirth.* Report of the Expert Maternity Group. London: HMSO.

Department of Health (1995). *Health Authorities Act.* London: HMSO.

Duerden, J.M. (1995). 'Audit of supervision of midwives in the North West Regional Health Authority'. Salford Royal Hospitals NHS Trust, p.20.

Flint, C. (1993). 'Big sister is watching you'. *Nursing Times* 89(46), November, pp.66–67.

English National Board for Nursing, Midwifery and Health Visiting (1992). *Preparation of Supervisors of Midwives.* Modules 1–4. London: ENB.

English National Board for Nursing, Midwifery and Health Visiting (1992). *Preparation for Supervisors of Midwives.* London: ENB.

English National Board for Nursing, Midwifery and Health Visiting (1995). *Developments in Midwifery Education and Practice – A Progress Report.* London: ENB.

Isherwood, K. (1988). 'Friend or watchdog?' *Nursing Times* 84(24), p.65.

Mayes, G. (1995). 'The challenge of changing childbirth'. Module 5, pp.33–41. London: ENB.

Statutory Instrument (1977). No. 1850. The Midwives (Qualifications of Supervisors).

Statutory Instrument (1993). No. 2106. The Nurses, Midwives and Health Visitors (Midwives Amendments) Rules Approval Order.

Steene, J. (1995). 'Supervision of midwives: proposed changes to the Midwives' Rules'. *British Journal of Midwifery,* Vol.3, No.9, September.

United Kingdom Central Council for Nursing, Midwifery and Health Visiting (1993). *Midwives Rules.* London: UKCC.

United Kingdom Central Council for Nursing, Midwifery and Health Visiting (1995). *Standards for Post-Registration Education and Practice.* London: UKCC.

The Protection
of the Public

CHAPTER FIVE

Supervision as a Public Service

> **Helen Lewison**
> is a former solicitor with extensive knowledge of Maternity services at national, regional and local levels. She has experience of project management and research through her work with the NCT, which she has been involved with since 1984 in many different capacities, including being an antenatal teacher. She became the National Chairwoman of the NCT in 1993/94 and was their representative on the Department of Health 'Changing Childbirth' Advisory Group. She was also a user representative on the UKCC Midwifery Committee from 1993-1995, where she submitted a paper on the supervision of midwives.

Protection of the public

Supervision of midwives evolved as one part of a framework for protecting the public from the perceived dangers of the handywomen who attended women in labour at the beginning of the twentieth century. The local supervising authorities (LSAs) are the bodies vested with the statutory power of exercising general supervision over midwives in accordance with the Midwives' Rules (UKCC, 1993), to report misconduct and to suspend midwives from practice (Nurses, Midwives and Health Visitors Act, 1979). These powers are exercised by supervisors appointed by LSAs under the provisions of the Midwives' Rules. It is a unique professional arrangement which has attracted criticism by some midwives and a few women over recent years. Does the public still need to be protected from poor standards of midwifery in this way? Whether or not supervision is the right mechanism, the arrangement will remain until the legislation is changed. Whilst the statutory requirements for supervision are in force, what are the nature and value of supervision for the childbearing public?

Supervision as an invisible element of maternity services

It has been observed that where supervision works well, it is invisible to the public (Page, 1995). Very little indeed has been written about women's experiences of supervision. The Journal of the Association for Improvements in Maternity Services (AIMS) is the only periodical for lay people which features supervision as an issue. Otherwise, the only time when supervision is mentioned in the lay press is in mother and baby magazines when a woman telling her story of arranging a home birth might mention a meeting with the supervisor of midwives. Indeed, the Midwife's Code of Practice (UKCC, 1994) is worded in such a way that it appears to be intended that it is always the midwife herself who maintains dialogue with a woman, even in the case of difficulties, whilst the supervisor remains in the background as a safety net for the woman and the midwife:

> 'You and your supervisor of midwives have a mutual responsibility for effective communication between you in order that any problems can be shared and a resolution achieved at the earliest opportunity' (paragraph 50).

Similarly, in the case of home birth:

> 'When the support of a medical practitioner is not available, you should discuss the situation in advance whenever possible with your supervisor of midwives, and agree and record appropriate arrangements to provide advice and support as necessary' (paragraph 55).

And:

> 'You and your supervisor of midwives, through your respective roles, should work towards a common aim of optimum care for mothers and babies' (paragraph 49).

Thus it is envisaged, and usually appears to be the case in practice, that the supervisor remains in the background, giving support 'as a colleague, counsellor and advisor' (paragraph 51). This is in tune with modern management theories such as those of Tom Peters (1982), which expound the principle that every staff member dealing with the public should be empowered to handle any situation that is likely to arise with a client without referral to higher authority.

One can compare this to the receipt of other services where one might, when dealing with an employee of an organization, see their superior. If the client asks to see a superior, this is usually because the client requires information or action beyond the powers or capabilities of the employee. This need not reflect badly on the employee provided they are fulfilling their job description - it can simply be a way for the client to access what they need from the organization more swiftly and it is likely to be regarded by the client as a reflection of the way the organization is managed. If, on the other hand, the transaction between the client and the employee is proceeding in a satisfactory manner, but the superior suddenly intervenes and takes over the dialogue with the client, or asks to see the client separately, this can disempower the employee and reduce the client's confidence in them.

Women's experiences of supervision

On the whole, women nowadays come into contact with supervisors of midwives only when a relationship with a midwife has gone badly wrong or when they make what are regarded by some local maternity services as unusual or unreasonable demands. It is more common for a supervisor to approach a woman than the other way round. For some years, it was the case that in some areas any request for a home birth merited a visit from the supervisor of midwives. The view of women so visited at that time appears to have been that their home was being looked over as a venue suitable for a home birth. Perhaps this was a hangover from the traditional duty of the supervisor to inspect midwives' homes and personal hygiene. In fact, 'the private residence of the mother and baby' are specifically excluded, and always have been, from the provisions concerning inspection of premises and equipment by supervisors (UKCC, 1993, paragraph 43).

In an antenatal class I taught in 1995, four of the eight women had planned to have their babies at home and, because I had been invited to write this chapter, I asked them whether they had been visited by a supervisor of midwives. Three had not been, although one of them planned to use a birthing pool. The woman who had been visited said that the visit had taken place not because she planned to use a birthing pool, but because she did not want to commit herself to coming out of the water for the delivery and preferred to keep her options open. (This visit by a supervisor was probably a result of the East Herts waterbirth case, where two midwives were suspended for allowing a woman to give birth under water, on which more below.) She reported the meeting as being a positive and helpful opportunity for herself and her partner to ask questions. She did not find the visit at all intimidating or threatening, and regarded it as the beginning of the professional care she was to receive for her home birth, with the midwives coming to her at home rather than asking her to meet them at the hospital.

Yet not all women find such meetings, or even the prospect of them, so positive. An AIMS member wrote in its Journal, 'The author might be surprised to know how many calls for help AIMS receives from women who are terrified by receiving just such an invitation when they request a home birth or waterbirth. They see themselves as under suspicion: women who have to be assessed, warned and watched by senior management, instead of normal healthy women making reasonable requests' (AIMS, 1995).

There have been many instances where either supervisors of midwives have tried to dissuade a mother from making what is perceived to be an unsuitable choice for birth or where the supervisor has failed to intervene in a situation where women have been unhappy with the care being given by their midwives (Beech, 1995). In the latter type of case, supervisors have failed in their duty to 'promote a positive working relationship which is conducive to maintaining and improving standards of practice and care' (UKCC 1994, paragraph 51). In the former situation, it is difficult to see with what authority a supervisor attempts to influence a woman, since none of the UKCC documents regulating midwifery practice makes provision for supervisors to intervene in a relationship between a woman and her midwife. It is more likely that the reason for dissuading the woman is that her wish to give birth at home runs counter to a local hospital policy designed to minimize the number of situations where risk of untoward incidents is increased and where the possibility of litigation is feared.

In such a case, the supervisor is in fact likely to be acting in her role as manager of midwifery services and senior employee of an NHS Trust rather than in her role as supervisor. It is just such actions which give rise to confusion between the two distinct roles of supervisor and manager and which cause midwives and women to call into question the nature and value of the role of the supervisor of midwives (Walton, 1995).

In the case of a visit by a supervisor to a woman's home, the intervention of a supervisor into the relationship between a woman and her midwife is very obvious. However, there are many more occasions in hospital where it is easier for supervisors to have direct contact with women and when, as a result, the role of the supervisor and the effect of her intervention on the relationship between the woman and the midwife caring for her are less clear. This is particularly the case on labour wards where so often health professionals enter delivery rooms without always asking permission, stating the reason for their visit or introducing themselves. Where it is easy from both a geographical and cultural point of view for a supervisor to enter a delivery room to speak to a woman or to check on her midwifery care, there is an increased risk that the supervisor will not stop to ask herself the following questions:

- in what role is she proposing to intervene - supervisor or manager or both?

- does she propose to make this explicit to the midwife and the woman?

- what effect is her intervention likely to have on the relationship between the woman and her midwife and, consequently, on the progress and management of the woman's labour and birth?

- is her intervention necessary?

Without such a process of self-examination being carried out by the supervisor, it is possible for a slippery slope to lead to erosion of the primary relationship between the woman and her midwife and a loss of autonomy for both.

Whom does supervision protect?

If supervision is truly to protect the public, why are women having babies not better informed about the role of the supervisor in helping maintain professional standards of midwifery?

The New Pregnancy Book (HEA, 1993) does not include the supervisor of midwives in its 'Who's Who' of professional staff involved in maternity services. Interestingly, though, given the experiences of some of the women who have been in touch with AIMS, it includes 'the local supervisor of midwives who is also usually head of maternity services at the local maternity or district general hospital' among the people and organizations 'you can also ask for information on your options from' (p. 29). Similarly, after saying that women desiring a home birth should 'first talk to your GP' it then recommends, 'If he or she cannot help... it's also a good idea to contact your local supervisor of midwives or the director of maternity services at the hospital. She will be able to arrange for a community midwife to call and discuss a home delivery' (p. 30). By contrast, the NCT leaflet on choices for childbirth (NCT, 1995) does not mention the supervisor. For women who wish to arrange a home birth it recommends, 'Your family doctor can arrange a home birth for you, but you don't need your doctor's permission. You can book a home birth directly with a midwife. Telephone your local hospital and ask for the community midwives'. And for a Domino Scheme birth: 'To find out if domino care is available in your area contact your local hospital and ask to speak to the community midwives'.

Whilst the maternity booklets of some enlightened maternity units inform women about how to make a complaint through the hospital system or by contacting their local community health council, it is rarely, if ever, suggested that they complain about the quality of midwifery care to the supervisor of midwives. The Patients's Charter for Maternity Services recommends the supervisor as a last resort for complaint:

'If you are dissatisfied with your NHS services:
If you have any concerns about your NHS services, please make them known to the people who provide those services - at your antenatal or postnatal clinic, GP's surgery or health centre, or at the hospital. If you are not satisfied with their response, contact the general manager or chief executive of the Family Health Services Authority or hospital, or the supervisor of midwives and they will let you know the ways your complaint can be handled' (Department of Health, 1994b, p.6).

This low public profile of the supervisor is likely to be appreciated by those midwives who consider that an individual should not fulfil both roles of supervisor and manager, but should the role of supervisor be better understood by the general public and should women be given more direct access to supervisors?

The question about whom the supervision is there to protect is relevant when considering the 1993 East Herts waterbirth case. Here, the woman involved was well-informed and planned to labour at home in a birthing pool and possibly to give birth in water if that felt right for her at the time. It was stated that it was the policy of the East Herts NHS Trust not to allow women to give birth in water on the grounds that they were not contracted with the health authority to provide this service. It was also the case that the community midwives were not trained to deliver babies born under water. However, there was in fact no way to prevent this happening without breaking the law:

- if the midwives left the woman unattended while she gave birth, they would be in breach of their professional duty;

- if they attempted to remove her from the birthing pool against her will, they would commit assault.

The arrangements for the birth were discussed by the woman, the midwives and the supervisor early on in pregnancy and the midwives had time to prepare themselves to care for the woman should she in fact give birth under water. However, the midwives 'omitted to ask the supervisor what she would advise should the woman refuse to move' (Beech, 1995) and, following the safe delivery of the baby under water, were suspended. The resulting publicity was particularly unfortunate, in three ways:

- it fuelled the argument that the supervision of midwives was an outmoded and oppressive system. This was at a time when both the UKCC and the ENB were striving to improve the practice of supervision: the UKCC by providing that supervisors should not take up office until suitably trained (UKCC, 1993, paragraph 44); the ENB by encouraging the use of its open learning pack on supervision (ENB, 1992).

- it resulted in several other NHS trusts adopting similar policies forbidding women either to give birth under water or to labour in water at all (personal communication, Mary Newburn, NCT). By doing this they were promulgating the fallacy that it was possible to prevent women from giving birth under water, even in their own homes and ignoring the widespread evidence (subsequently formally collected by the National Perinatal Epidemiology Unit) that waterbirths were safe provided that certain straightforward precautions were undertaken (Alderdice et al, 1995).

- it created the impression that women were wantonly putting their babies' lives at risk by indulging in unusual birthing practices at a time when the recent publication of 'Changing Childbirth' (Department of Health, 1993) was encouraging changes in maternity services aimed to promote women's choice and control in relation to their care.

There have been many other cases where supervisors' actions in relation to other hospital policies, equally outdated and lacking an evidence base, have in effect protected not the public, but rather:

- midwives who have not met their statutory obligation to acquire new skills required by their practice (UKCC, 1994, paragraph 23). For example, where a supervisor attempts to dissuade a woman from choosing a home birth because the community midwives have not been trained to suture the perineum or put up an intravenous drip.

- GPs who have refused to support women's requests for a home birth in contravention of the clear government statement that:

'Where a woman wants a home birth and her GP does not wish, for whatever reason, to provide care, the GP is required to help her make other arrangements, if she so wishes, for example, by referring her to another GP or to the supervisor of midwives. The latter will, if necessary, arrange for a midwife to provide the care that is needed without the involvement of a GP' (Department of Health, 1992, paragraph 2.13.3).

Here, by implication, any supervisor who does not ensure that GPs know how to contact her, is colluding with GPs unwilling to accede to women's requests for a home birth.

- obstetricians who persist in outdated practices and allow policies not based on evidence to determine maternity care given by all staff in a unit, including midwives. The recent report of the Clinical Standards Advisory Group (Department of Health, 1995) is full of examples of practice in maternity units all over the country where midwives, by giving evidence-based care such as not directing women to push in the second stage of labour, were in fact in breach of outdated protocols for care in labour. In theory, at least, this leaves maternity units vulnerable to litigation. In these cases, it could be argued that the supervisors were in breach of paragraph 52 of The Midwife's Code of Practice:

'Supervisors of midwives should ensure that effective communication links exist between themselves, LSAs, those engaged in determining health service policy and medical staff in order that relevant issues are appropriately addressed and resolved'.

- themselves, in cases where their own deficiencies are projected on to the midwives to whom they are statutorily required to give 'support as a colleague, counsellor and advisor. This should be developed in order to promote a positive working relationship which is conducive to maintaining and improving standards of practice and care' (UKCC, 1994, paragraph 51).

The potential value of the supervisor to women using maternity services

The International Code of Ethics for Midwives (ICM, 1993) 'makes public the goals, values and morals of those who call themselves midwives' (p.11). Notably, it gives 'Midwifery Relationships' as the title of its first section. The Midwife's Code of Practice also identifies supportive relationships and communication as important elements in the functioning of the supervisor's role, by saying:

'A key and important aspect of this supervisory function is that it enables this process [of effective communication]' (paragraph 50) and

'This [support] should be developed in order to promote a positive working relationship which is conducive to maintaining and improving standards of practice and care' (paragraph 51).

It is therefore possible to take each of the six articles contained in the Midwifery Relationships section of the International Code in turn and examine the potential for the supervisor's role in promoting good communication and relationships with both women and midwives.

'a. Midwives respect a woman's informed right of choice and promote the woman's acceptance of responsibility for the outcomes of her choices.'

Since the adoption of 'Changing Childbirth' as government policy in January 1994 (Department of Health, 1994a), there has been anecdotal evidence that some midwives have interpreted the report's emphasis on choice as meaning that women should be left to make all the choices with no support. This attitude disregards the fact that women have been discouraged for so long from taking control and making choices in relation to so many aspects of their lives, that for some it is a new skill which cannot be learned overnight. Similarly, many midwives have not been trained to facilitate informed decision-making by women and also have new skills of active listening and clear information-giving to learn. This is exactly the sort of area that could be addressed by a midwife in consultation with her supervisor with a view to identifying possible ways of meeting her training needs.

The Midwife's Code of Practice gives the supervisor a distinct role in supporting a midwife when a mother rejects her advice in relation to the type of care she wishes to have, with the exhortation to the midwife to 'continue to give unbiased care to the best of your ability, seeking peer support as necessary' (paragraph 17). Similarly, where a mother refuses the medical assistance required by a midwife, the midwife is required to 'consult as soon as possible with your supervisor of midwives, making a detailed record of the circumstances and action taken' (paragraph 18). In neither case does the code provide that the supervisor should intervene personally; instead, it is implied that the supervisor should be available for advice and to support the midwife, thus enabling the midwife to conform to the definition, 'Each midwife as a practitioner of midwifery is accountable for her own practice in whatever environment she practises' (UKCC, 1994, paragraph 2).

'b. Midwives work with women, supporting their right to participate actively in decisions about their care, and empowering women to speak for themselves on issues affecting the health of women and their families in their culture/society.'

If women are to be empowered to make their own decisions and to voice their own opinions in relation to childbirth, midwives themselves have to be empowered in order to pass on to the women for whom they care the knowledge and the confidence to speak up for themselves. Supervisors can empower midwives by helping them build their knowledge and confidence through reflective practice. Too often, women have become involved in work as consumer representatives through negative experiences and this can sometimes colour the tone of their contributions to debate and alienate the professionals who need to be influenced. How different things might be if women were inspired by their good experiences of maternity care to help improve services for all women having babies.

'c. Midwives, together with women, work with policy and funding agencies to define women's needs for health services and to ensure that resources are fairly allocated considering priorities and availability.'

The obvious forum for this activity to take place is the Maternity Services Liaison Committee (Department of Health,1993, paras 3.2.3 and 4.2.2) which, if properly constituted, should have representation from both purchasers and providers of maternity care as well as representatives of service users and other stakeholders (Lewison, 1994). It is likely that many of the midwives nominated to serve on Maternity Services Liaison Committees will be supervisors and will be in a position to influence strategic and policy decisions in relation to maternity services, well-informed by their working relationships with the midwives they supervise and, possibly, by the services they manage. Through both formal and informal working relationships with consumer representatives on Maternity Services Liaison Committees, there is potential for each to understand each other's point of view and find ways of helping to make the provision of services acceptable to both women and midwives.

The NCT has received reports of this role of allocating resources being used rather negatively. Midwives in some areas have complained that it is well-educated, articulate NCT members who find out about scarce resources such as Domino births and take midwives away from less affluent women who have a greater need for their services (Lewison, 1993). It is for supervisors to take the lead in campaigning for better midwifery provision for all women and to discourage negative reports of this kind. Such reports give rise to questions such as, 'Why is information about all maternity care options not available to all women?' and, 'What evidence is there that socio-economic criteria are the only way of determining how much midwifery care different women should receive?'

'd. Midwives support and sustain each other in their professional roles, and actively nurture their own and others' sense of self-worth.'

Midwives are more likely to use peer support as a professional tool if this is modelled by supervisors in their relations both with each other and with midwives. Again, midwives used to promoting each other's self-esteem are likely to do the same with the women they care for. One effective model for peer support is that used by NCT antenatal teachers and breastfeeding counsellors who meet on a regular basis to share work experiences and problems in a safe, non-judgmental atmosphere with the aim of learning from reflection and each other's ideas and ways of approaching different situations. Where the support of peers is insufficient, antenatal and breastfeeding tutors are available for further support. Interestingly, where a problem with an antenatal teacher or breastfeeding counsellor is reported by a client, it would be the tutor who would be charged with investigating what happened and recommending further action. Whilst midwives use midwifery forums and journal clubs to share new knowledge, it appears to be less common for them to meet in informal groups with their peers in order to facilitate reflective practice. Supervisors might have a role in encouraging these meetings and negotiating with management time out from work for this purpose.

> **'e. Midwives work with other health professionals, consulting and referring as necessary when the woman's need for care exceeds the competencies of the midwife.'**
>
> There is a delicate balance to be maintained between the midwife extending her competencies as her growing experience, research and women's choices determine, and having a clear idea of her professional and personal boundaries so that she refers women to the care of other professionals appropriately. This is recognized in The Midwife's Code of Practice (paragraph 15). The supervisor has a statutory responsibility for supporting midwives both in extending their skills (UKCC, 1994, paragraph 23) and in receiving notification from midwives about 'any deviation from the norm' even when a midwife has called 'to her assistance a registered medical practitioner' (UKCC, 1993, paragraph 40 (1)).
>
> The Midwife's Code of Practice recognizes the importance of 'mutual recognition of the respective roles of midwives and registered medical practitioners and those others who may participate in the care of mothers and babies. Such mutual respect should enhance care and practice must be based upon agreed standards to ensure effective communication and co-operation in care' (paragraph 16). I would suggest that supervisors also have a role in promoting these agreed standards and mutual recognition and respect through ongoing work both with midwives and with members of all other professional groups involved in maternity care.

> **'f. Midwives recognize the human interdependence within their field of practice and actively seek to resolve inherent conflicts.'**
>
> There will be times when conflict will occur between midwives and members of other professional groups; midwives and women; midwives and supervisors; midwives and midwives. Supervisors are well placed and should have sufficient experience and training to facilitate the resolution of such conflicts.

Conclusion

Changing the relationship between supervisors of midwives and women using the maternity services needs to be thought about very carefully.

At present, as demonstrated previously, the positive presence of the supervisor in the background to the relationship between the woman and her midwife empowers the midwife to enable the woman to build up her knowledge of and confidence in the process of pregnancy and birth. The woman can then make informed choices and communicate them to the midwife. If these choices require an extension of the midwife's competencies, sensitive and skilful supervision can enable the midwife to increase her own skills and experience through meeting the woman's needs: a win-win situation in the language of management.

I would therefore recommend that women have more direct access to midwives, preferably their named midwife (Department of Health, 1994b) but not to supervisors of midwives. Furthermore, I would invite supervisors of midwives to think very carefully about the occasions on which, and the manner in which, they intervene in the primary relationship between a woman and her midwife. When it appears that intervention is necessary, a useful question for supervisors to ask themselves might be, 'Who am I aiming to protect by making this visit or telephone call?' One aspect of the supervisor's role which merits little attention, and which has great potential if developed, is that of leadership. In any field where rapid, radical change is occurring, strong leadership informed by vision and objectivity is essential. Supervisors are ideally placed to give midwives the leadership they require in order that women having babies can benefit from super-vision (ARM, 1995).

References

AIMS (1995). 'Emily's choice and the ethics of waterbirth'. *AIMS Journal* 7:1.

Alderdice, F. et al. (1995). 'Labour and birth in water in England and Wales'. *British Medical Journal*, Vol. 310, p.837.

Association of Radical Midwives (1995). *Super-vision. Consensus Conference Proceedings*. Hale: Books for Midwives Press.

Beech, B.L. (1995). 'The consumer view in association of radical midwives' in ARM (Ed). *Super-vision. Consensus Conference Proceedings*. Hale: Books for Midwives Press.

Department of Health (1992). *Maternity Services*. Government Response to the Second Report from the Health Committee, Session 1991-92. London: HMSO.

Department of Health (1993). *Changing Childbirth*. The Report of the Expert Maternity Group. London: HMSO.

Department of Health (1994a). *NHS Executive Letter Woman-centred Maternity Services*. 24 January EL(94)9.

Department of Health (1994b). *Patient's Charter*. Maternity Services. London: HMSO.

Department of Health (1995). *Clinical Standards Advisory Group: Women in Normal Labour*. London: HMSO.

ENB (1992). *Preparation of Supervisors of Midwives: An Open Learning Programme*. London: ENB.

Health Education Authority (1993). *New Pregnancy Book*. London: HMSO.

International Confederation of Midwives (1993). *International Code of Ethics for Midwives*. London: ICM.

Lewison, H. (1993). 'Report on continuity of care survey from replies to 1992 registration forms from NCT members sitting on outside bodies'. Unpublished.

Lewison, H. (1994). *Maternity Services Liaison Committees. A Forum for Change*. Greater London Association of Community Health Councils and National Childbirth Trust, London.

National Childbirth Trust (1995). *Where Should I have My Baby? Your Choices for Childbirth*. London: NCT.

Page, S. (1995). Letter. *Midwives* 108:1, 290 July pp.228-9.

Peters, T.J., Waterman, R.H. (1982). *In Search of Excellence: Lessons from America's Best Run Companies*. New York: Harper & Row.

UKCC (1993). *Midwives Rules*. London: UKCC.

UKCC (1994). *The Midwife's Code of Practice*. London: UKCC.

Walton, I. (1995). 'Conflicts in supervision of midwives' in Association of Radical Midwives (Ed). *Super-vision. Consensus Conference Proceedings*. Hale: Books for Midwives Press.

Examples of
Good Practice

CHAPTER SIX

Care for the Carers in Exeter

Kate Caldwell RGN, RM

After working in London for 20 years in both hospital and community posts, Kate Caldwell became Director of Midwifery Sevices in Exeter in 1990. Here she has implemented a successful team midwifery scheme in the hospital and now in the community. She also has represented the RCM on various commitees and is a member of the Council and the RCM English Board, as well as the ENB Professional Midwifery Advisory Group.

I believe supervision is one of the greatest strengths for the profession of midwifery. Such a bold statement needs to be justified. This chapter sets out to demonstrate how valuable the strength of supervision has become in Exeter. The role of the supervisor of midwives was developed in 1902 and has been evolving ever since. In 1979, the Nurses, Midwives, and Health Visitors Act was passed and the Midwives Rules and the role of the supervisor were reassessed. In 1992, the development of the ENB distance learning training pack 'Preparation of Supervisors of Midwives' (ENB, 1992) helped supervisors understand the work and role better. This is of support, professional development and assessment of midwives professional competence, all of which has brought the quality of midwifery to a level that I believe the country can be proud of.

The role of the supervisor is protected in statute (HMSO, 1979). As midwifery has developed and the expectations and demands of mothers have increased, so the needs of midwives have altered. Midwifery is now taught at diploma or degree level. Team midwifery and case load practice have developed in various forms around the country (Flint, 1993; Page, 1995). These changes have required considerable adjustment for midwives. Let us look at some of these changes.

The National Health Service reforms, though not obviously affecting clinical midwifery as the practice changes have done, have placed other pressures on the carers. Senior midwifery managers have had to adapt to the requirements put on them by Trusts, such as reductions in managerial staff, working to contract levels, working within more stringent budgets and constant review of skill mix. 'Changing Childbirth' (Department of Health, 1993) in giving indicators of success has put professional practice pressures on providers to adapt their organizations.

Since the first NHS provider trusts came into being, the agenda for provision of care has changed enormously.

Most midwives are women and have in the past worked because they enjoyed it, were fulfilled by the work and it suited them to do so. During the recent years of recession the work ethos has changed. More midwives are now in the position of needing to earn more money as the main family wage earner (Haralambos, 1995). This has added another pressure on midwives lives already burdened with changes in practice.

Midwives do not wish to, and indeed should not, work without days off. They cannot and should not be expected to commit their lives only to their work on a long term basis. Evidence has shown (Wheeler and Riding, 1994) that long work hours can cause burn out and exhaustion leading to the mistakes that good supervision is trying to avoid.

The erosion of extended families in British society (Central Statistical Office, 1995) and the increase in divorce and single parent families has meant that midwives have had to develop their skills in social work, counselling and family support (OPCS, 1993). These skills were always there to a certain extent but social trends have created a need in some cases to give more commitment and that has created more personal pressure on the midwives which needs to be recognized by the supervisor.

Following the publication of 'Changing Childbirth' (Department of Health,1993) maternity departments without teams had a new challenging aspect of care to be addressed. Midwives who had worked in exclusive areas of practice were asked to join teams, sometimes having to work in areas in which they had not worked for some considerable time. The development of teams of midwives meant that sometimes midwives were working with colleagues they neither liked nor felt empathy with. Midwives who were unfamiliar with home deliveries, due to lack of experience, needed to develop those skills and possibly more alarming to them, learn to take on the different role and responsibility of a community midwife.

There is a cascade of pressures from midwife managers, themselves often feeling threatened by the changes in patterns of care and the needs of the Health Service Trusts trying to keep within budget. This can filter down to all staff within the units and community. Professional development, discussion and advice is needed to provide a safety net. To maintain good professional practice the statute for supervision is therefore essential.

Midwifery supervision should be a positive and supportive experience enjoyed by the midwife and supervisor alike. It is not about management, but is about professional practice development and recognizing strengths and weaknesses and seeing what changes are needed by the midwife in her practice. Supervision is a professional relationship between the nominated, named supervisor and the midwife which encompasses equal commitment, open and honest discussions and joint responsibility for the actions resulting from the supervision. Safe care for women is achieved by a midwife having professional support from her supervisor, and the skill of how to reflect on her practice, assess her work and therefore expand her knowledge.

Although supervision needs a certain formality and commitment it also needs an openness and availability. A relationship of trust, honesty and openness needs to be maintained. In the next part of this chapter I will give some practical ways of providing this support based on the Exeter model.

In Exeter each midwife has a named supervisor. This supervisor is allocated but all midwives are free to approach another either permanently or for advice and support at any time.

There is the opportunity for fairly formal supervision meetings, at least annually, to discuss the way forward on some of the objectives of a professional nature identified during performance appraisal undertaken by the appraiser and appraisee.

Most supervision is on a one-to-one basis, although peer group or discussion groups are sometimes valuable. A supervisor needs to be readily available and an on-call rota is available to all staff. To enable accessibility, individual supervisors have an open door style during their working hours.

Supervision focuses on activity specific to midwifery practice. In Exeter we have developed a programme called 'Care for the Carers' which complements the more formal and recognized supervision. The programme has been built on the following philosophy.

Philosophy

- Staff have the right to be treated with respect as intelligent, capable and equal human beings.
- Organizational attitude is crucial to success. Staff have permission to acknowledge stress without fear of stigma and reprisals.
- Time, effort and money is invested into the well-being of each individual.
- By showing a caring attitude, individuals will feel better about themselves, their work will be enriched and the health of the total organization will be improved.

The philosophy behind the scheme is to recognize the difficulties that staff have in their professional and private lives whilst continuing to provide the level of care for their clients that is expected of them.

A nurse counsellor is employed full time to support and train staff with the counselling and bereavement issues which arise. She is there to support the midwife for any mother needing more counselling input than an individual midwife may be able to give. The nurse counsellor holds regular training sessions on counselling, bereavement and grief. There is also a completely confidential service of counselling and counselling supervision available for any staff who wish to use it. This ensures that all staff who have a high counselling input in their daily work have access to a supervisor to discuss case issues .

It is crucial that midwives develop a personal sense of self awareness to enable each individual to identify her own stress, its effects on her and its effects on others. Midwives need to feel positive about themselves and the team they work in. Positive thoughts about improving the service are more conducive to good teamwork than negative thoughts about how to survive. To support midwives in this, a psychotherapist is employed on a regular basis to work on team building and general coping skills. This is often in the form of workshops allowing groups to explore issues within a safe and supportive environment and thereby to develop personal and team strategies.

To encourage a feeling of well being and a sense of being valued massage is available free of charge to staff twice a month. Staff trained in therapeutic massage are able to set aside time each month to give their colleagues massage. To be able to take 20 minutes 'time out' in their working day ensures midwives positively acknowledge their need to care for themselves.

Another important aspect of valuing and being valued is provided by social events. Two main parties are held during working time, one on Pancake day and the other a barbecue which is held in the summer, both to acknowledge the importance of taking time out and taking time for oneself and colleagues.

These social events are now an accepted norm. Other events have been adopted by individual teams both on and off duty to continue to enhance the support and care given by all staff to one another.

More and more ethical dilemmas continue to arise. The development of antenatal testing and diagnosis, the greater scope in sub fertility care and a higher survival rate of premature babies at even lower gestational ages gives rise for concern. Ethical discussion groups which include neonatal nurses and gynaecology staff are held to share some of the dilemmas midwives find themselves in and to search for personal answers that individuals can come to terms with and to be able to understand how colleagues are coping with dilemmas.

All midwives know they have permission to express their stress and their concerns and know they have many varied forms of support from which they can find some help to suit their needs.

Statutory supervision is there for all but the other provision of care is for those who want it, need it or value of it.

Midwifery supervision is primarily about support for professional competence and development (ENB, 1992). The 'Care for the Carers' scheme is about development of self, self awareness and having permission to acknowledge problems, and/or stress and do something about it. The package gives many support mechanisms to the staff to help them feel valued and have opportunities to recognize ways of self preservation for work and home.

With these extra skills communication with mothers and colleagues is improved, offering a higher quality of care and a greater unity in the teams.

Evaluation of the 'Care for the Carers' scheme has been carried out. Amongst the findings were that the sickness rate for staff in the Maternity Department is between two and four per cent per annum which is low when compared with statistics from other departments. The maternity services were evaluated using the Office of Population Censuses and Surveys 'Women's Experience in Maternity Care' (OPCS, 1989) and the mother's perception of the quality of care has been excellent and this would appear to be as a result of midwives being able to deliver excellent care because they themselves are cared for (Welsh et al., 1993).

The take up of the 'Care for the Carers' scheme has been good. There is little doubt that the commitment and enthusiasm of the midwives is very real and stimulating to the department and teams. Several research projects and audits have been initiated by

---

Menu of care for the carers
Wide range to allow for individual choice

Appetiser
Awakens the jaded palate
Knowing what is available
Experiencing care
Hearing from others
Permission to accept care

Starter
Sets the scene for a good meal
Personal time

Self Awareness	Supervision
Self Development	Group Work
Professional Training	Appraisals
Personal Counselling	Books

Main Course
Range of different flavours originally presented
Patient contact issues
Sharing patients, with other disciplines
Team building and working
Time
Debriefing
Permission to ask for help
Mentors/Facilitators

Dessert
The part of the meal that some have saved up for... and others consider almost sinful
What can we give to and accept from others
Praise
Value
Recognition
Thanks

Wine List
Different types to flow throughout
Communication

Coffee
Genuine ground type, not the instant variety
The extras that make all the difference
Massage
Relaxation tapes
Meditation

Liqueur
Something extra

N.A.S.S.

Fig. 6.1: Menu of care for carers
(published courtesy of Modern Midwife)

staff to improve the care that is provided. Such projects are evidence of the high levels of energy and enthusiasm which abound in the unit.

The programme has been illustrated in the form of a menu displayed in the unit as an enjoyable reminder to staff of the programme (see opposite).

Conclusion

Midwifery supervision is exciting. It challenges practice. It ensures safe practice. It is governed by statute.

When linked with a 'Care for the Carers' programme that is confidential, safe and individually focused, supervision becomes one of the greatest strengths for the midwifery profession hence my bold statement at the beginning of this chapter.

References

Caldwell, K., Derbyshire, F., Elworthy, J., Smith, G. (1995). 'Food for thought; a menu for supervision'. *Modern Midwife*.

Central Statistical Office (1995). *Social Trends*. London: HMSO.

Department of Health (1993). *Changing Childbirth*. London: HMSO.

English National Board (1992). *Preparation of Supervisors of Midwives*. London: ENB.

Flint, C. (1993). *Midwifery Teams and Caseloads*. Oxford: Butterworth-Heinemann.

Haralambos, M., Holborn, M. (1995). *Sociology: Themes and Perspectives*. Collins Educational.

Her Majesty's Stationery Office (1979). *Nurses, Midwives and Health Visitors Act 1989*. London: HMSO.

Foster, K., Jackson, B., Thomas, M., Hunter, P. (1993). *Office of Population, Censuses and Surveys*. General Household Survey.

Page, L. (1995). *Effective Group Practice in Midwifery*. Oxford: Blackwell Science.

Welsh, L., Caldwell, K., Caves, R. (1993). *Womens Experience of Maternity Services*. Exeter Health Authority.

Welsh, L. (1995). *Women's Experience of Maternity Care in Honiton, Okehampton, Tiverton and Heavitree Hospitals*. Exeter and North Devon Health Authority.

Wheeler, H., Riding, R. (1994). 'Occupation stress in general nurses and midwives'. *British Journal of Nursing*, Vol. 3, No 10.

CHAPTER SEVEN

Enabling Midwives to Practice Better

Rosemary Johnson RN, RM
became Maternity Services Manager at the Southmead NHS Trust, Bristol in September 1993. She previously worked as both a hospital and community midwife in Reading and then in Bristol, where she became a Supervisor of Midwives in 1988. Here she developed a keen interest in midwifery management, especially in developing caseload audit tools and the role of the midwife.

Introduction

This chapter is written in the light of eight years experience as a supervisor of midwives during which time three different posts were held both in community and hospital management. My current post as Maternity Services Manager at Southmead NHS Trust combines general management with a professional advisory role. Southmead Maternity Services provides care to approximately 5500 women and their families each year. Approximately 200 midwives notify their intention to practice annually, practising in hospital, community, neonatal intensive care, and midwifery teaching. This provides a variety of supervisory experience.

Supervisors potentially have complex and sometimes contradictory roles, being required to be 'concerned with the safety of practice and care' and 'a support, colleague and advisor' (UKCC, 1994) whilst also being the woman's advocate (ENB, 1994). The supervisor may face problems similar to those described by Schon (1990):

> 'In the varied topography of professional practice, there is a high, hard ground overlooking a swamp. On the high ground, manageable problems lend themselves to solution through the application of research based theory and technique. In the swampy lowland, messy, confusing problems defy technical solution' (p.3).

Such 'swampy' issues require professional skill to resolve as no ready made text book solutions are available. A description is, however, given of some of the processes, illustrated by examples, which have been found helpful in providing general supervision.

Effective supervision should be intimately involved with the local situation, able to initiate and manage change whilst being able to react swiftly to situations that arise. This chapter cannot provide a blue print for successful supervision but aims to challenge the reader to review the practice of supervision in their local situation giving illustrations that they may wish to consider applying. Some concepts are adapted from ideas and experience gained from general management, whilst others are copied and adapted from ideas that are common in society and commerce. The examples relate to midwifery supervision within the NHS. Independent midwifery practice and care contracted to midwifery group practices may become more common in future, particularly if such schemes are cost effective. Such radical changes will require further development within the process and administration of midwifery supervision, however the principles of good practice should remain unchanged.

The majority of examples are based on an 'action learning' circle, of which there are numerous models. Kolb's model of Action Research and Experiential Learning (1984) describes a learning circle consisting of experience, observations, formation of concepts and testing. Such a simple model is unable to represent the emotion and dynamics that are integral to learning particularly when the 'experience' involves serious professional issues that have long standing consequences. Using this approach has, however, led the supervisory team to view supervision as a process that involves continual development, learning, regular review and change.

Minztberg (1973) observed managers working and discovered that their role was complex and described the manager's job in terms of various roles derived from the bestowed formal authority. These roles are described as interpersonal, informational and decisional. The role of the supervisor, although a professional activity, bears many resemblances to those of managers, requiring a balancing of demands, choices and constraints (Stewart, 1982). Supervisors have demands made of them (accountabilities), choices to make about the way they fulfil their role, and constraints (often insufficient time but possibly political constraints driven by other roles they have in the organization). Supervisors may find it helpful to read general management texts to enhance their understanding of how complex roles are addressed in other settings.

General supervision
Selecting and nominating supervisors
Previously a specific midwifery post, the managerial or clinical grade, and the nomination of that midwife as a supervisor have often been linked. Now a variety of other methods are also being used to select midwives for nomination as a supervisor. Leaving aside debates which argue against a system that might link a specific post with a supervisory role, where this system exists, consideration needs to be given to the job description and personal specification to ensure that sufficient weight is given to the midwifery supervision element of the post. Existing supervisors should negotiate with the service manager their recommendations regarding the job description and personal specification of such posts. Where nomination as a supervisor is not linked to a specific post, some areas ask for expressions of interest from midwives who are then interviewed, selected and nominated according to their merit. These systems of nomination do not have to exclude each other, particularly if some supervisors hold managerial posts whilst others are clinically

based. Whichever system of nomination is adopted, the focus may rightly be directed on the individual accountability of each supervisor within a non hierarchical professional structure. A totally individualistic approach to midwifery supervision, concentrating solely on the duties and responsibilities of individual supervisors (ENB, 1994) may however deny the profession the benefits that a team approach can provide.

Developing a team approach

A team approach for tackling complex management problems requiring co-ordination of individual functions or tasks has become common place within general management (Kakabadse, Ludlow and Vinnicombe, 1988). Accepting the philosophy that a team approach could be effective at producing management solutions, it was considered that a similar approach might enhance midwifery supervision and consequently a supervisory team has been developed at Southmead. The team wanted to be equipped to provide a better framework for general midwifery supervision and a fuller range of professional advice, particularly during the transition of midwifery roles associated with the implementation of 'Changing Childbirth' (Department of Health, 1993). Consideration was given to the areas of midwifery practice at Southmead that warranted specific expertise within the supervisory team and the following broad aspects of midwifery practice were identified:

- Acute clinical care
- Antenatal care
- Community care
- Management
- Midwifery teaching
- Specialist neonatal care
- Practice development
- Research.

The supervisors acknowledged that they could not realistically maintain consistent competency in every area of practice. Taking into account the skill mix within the existing team, midwives with specialist neonatal and teaching experience were required and two such midwives were subsequently nominated. If this approach to nomination is adopted, a generic personal specification for supervisors of midwives is no longer appropriate as the personal specification must reflect the specific requirements of the team at a given time. This will depend on the skill mix within the team and its changing priorities and objectives.

Apart from the professional skills required by the team, consideration was given to how individuals function in teams, effecting the overall team success (Belbin, 1981). Using questionnaires based on Belbin's research, each supervisor completed a self analysis questionnaire. This enabled them to recognize their primary and secondary role preference within a team. Undertaking the Belbin team analysis helped the team to identify where there might be a natural lack in the team functioning (our team lacked a 'finisher') and to value individual difference. The totally 'pragmatic' supervisor (or company worker) can be irritated by the strategist (or monitor evaluator) within the group. However an understanding of group dynamics can enhance team functioning and reduce team tension (Mottram, 1982).

Having adopted this team approach, supervisors wished to raise the profile of midwifery supervision and to make supervision more accessible. A small booklet was produced giving details of all the supervisors special interests, expertise and contact information.

Rosemary Johnson

Present post - Maternity Services Manager

Professional interests
- Professional development
- Breastfeeding
- Policy making and its effect on midwifery practice
- Midwifery supervision

Other interests
- Risk management in maternity care
- Ethics and maternity care (currently undertaking M.Sc. Management Development and Social Responsibility)
- Developing new models of maternity care
- Contracting and maternity services

Areas of expertise
- Litigation and complaints procedures
- Breastfeeding advice
- All aspects of community midwifery and community aspects of care
- Home births
- Liaison with other professions/agencies especially medical staff

Contact information
Contact via midwifery office, appointments available via my secretary. If urgent contact via pager (number ....) to speak to the 'on call' supervisor (available 24 hours).

Fig. 7.1: Example of supervisors' details

This information booklet was circulated to all midwives on receipt of their notification of intention to practice. It was hoped that this would enable a more informed choice for midwives when selecting a named supervisor, seeking advice on a particular issue or professional development advice.

What is supervision for?

Supervisors may respond with a definition related to the inception of midwifery supervision in the 1902 Act, the statutory nature of supervision, protection of the public and their supportive role to midwives. All of this is of course correct and such general statements provide a flavour of what supervision should be achieving. To be effective however, more detailed planning is required if high ideals are to be translated into good practice in the 'swampy lowland'. A key question for the team was 'what is supervision *really* for at Southmead'. Supervisors considered the question in depth to determine the immediate local midwifery practice needs. Supervisors required information to enable them to answer this question and following annual reviews of midwives the supervisor completed an anonymous pro forma. This provided broad details of the issues or problems that had been identified during each interview. The information was entered onto a data base, providing a detailed profile of supervisory issues and enabled supervisors to prioritise and plan supervisory activities for the next year.

Issue	Plan
A concern by midwives that they lack experience in a community setting while others require an update in acute skills.	A programme of midwifery experience schemes involving job swaps.
Difficulties with record keeping due to the style of the maternity records.	Establish a multidisciplinary working group to revise the maternity records.

Fig. 7.2: Supervisory issues and planning

The objectives for supervision during the year then formed part of the *supervisory strategy* which formed an integral part of the Maternity Services Strategy. Issues common to a large number of midwives were noted and a plan for resolving the practice issues was devised on a group rather than an individual level. Having the benefit of a clear strategic direction, supervisors could focus their energy on the identified and agreed priorities. The supervisors then discussed the best means of resolving these issues, and the plan was agreed by the Service Manager (who when wearing a managerial hat has to be assured of other matters e.g. budget, efficiency, the effect on overall service provision etc). Having established the strategic direction a 'Theme for the Year' was decided and advertised to midwives e.g. Empowering Midwives. There are a number of ways that strategy formation can be approached and recommended further reading is 'Exploring Corporate Strategy' by Johnson and Scholes (1993).

A business planning approach to supervision

A business planning approach can be appropriate to facilitate improvements in midwifery practice. A number of approaches to business planning exist and one of these can easily be adapted to midwifery supervision. Recommended further reading is 'The Strategy Process: Concepts, Contexts, Cases' (Mintzberg and Quinn, 1991).

For example a 'SWOT' analysis was undertaken at Southmead. This involves examining the internal 'Strengths, Weaknesses, Opportunities and Threats' to midwifery practice.

Strengths	Stable work force of midwives Good basic skills base demonstrated by audit
Weaknesses	A number of influential midwives generally resistant to change A number of clinical practices not research based
Opportunities	Effective 'Practice Development Group' Many midwives enthusiastic to provide integrated hospital and community midwifery care
Threats	Some midwives reluctant to practice autonomously Frustration amongst midwives that the LHA has no additional money to fund the implementation of 'Changing Childbirth'.

Fig. 7.3: A 'SWOT' analysis

An analysis was also undertaken of external factors e.g. demographic changes, economic trends, relationships with other service providers, relationships with key stake holders (the women and their families), changing expectations of society, etc. This is also described as a PEST analysis looking at the Political, Environmental, Social and Technological changes that can potentially affect a business or service. Given the information obtained from the SWOT and PEST analyses, the supervisors were able to refine the supervisory strategy. They also had the advantage of having the basis of a full business case for submission to the Trust. When approaching senior managers for development funding relating to clinical developments or changes in care provision, it is essential to use language which is familiar to business and finance managers and to demonstrate that an acceptable methodology has been used.

The supervisory team and networking

Supervisors need to learn from situations but many situations are fortunately rare and may only be experienced once during a supervisory career. Networking with colleagues is vital to disseminate learning and obtain the best advice through collaboration. Sharing information also provides a learning environment for recently nominated supervisors. Some supervisors may find themselves in an isolated position either through geographical constraints, or because of power difference (attributable to employment posts) between themselves and other supervisors. This will limit the supervisory experience of the whole team. Southmead has tried to address these issues by having regular team meetings, which include an open invitation to supervisors working in isolation in the nearby locality. The meetings are very informal and every attempt is made to facilitate a 'team' rather than a structured or 'hierarchical' meeting. Midwives undertaking the supervisors preparation course are invited to attend (irrespective of whether they have been nominated as a supervisor) enabling them to gain both a theoretical and practice-based perspective of supervision. This functioning supervisory team has enabled supervisors to be more influential in the midwifery environment whilst providing welcome mutual support.

Risk management

Supervision may be viewed purely as a 'one to one' professional activity but some situations affect all midwives practising in the area. Midwifery supervision can be most effective in such scenarios by ensuring that the supervisory team utilize their professional knowledge to lead the policy and guideline process. This proactive approach to supervision will provide a safer practice environment and interacts well with 'clinical risk management' systems. Southmead are currently implementing such a system and the maternity service has volunteered to be the pilot site! Supervisors will be able to use the risk management data base to further inform the 'focus' of their supervisory activities as well as having rapid and easy access to reports of all maternity incidents. This has the potential for enhancing midwifery practice whilst raising the profile of midwifery supervision.

Supervision and the practice environment.

The implementation of 'Changing Childbirth' (Department of Health, 1993) and the concept of integrated care is radically affecting the practice environment at Southmead. If supervision is being effective, this change should raise new challenges for supervisors.

One such example has been the introduction and audit of 'midwife bookings'. The hospital had previously only provided hospital based care under the authority of a consultant obstetrician or general practitioner. The implementation of midwife bookings required supervisors to develop policy and guidelines which appropriately reflected the role of the midwife practising normal midwifery. Small focus groups were formed so that midwives could discuss and formulate the guidelines for their clinical area. Each group was facilitated by a supervisor of midwives and draft guidelines were then circulated widely to midwives and medical staff for comment.

All community based midwives were provided with an individual copy of the finalized policy and guidelines (copies are readily available in the hospital to all other midwives). Change rarely runs smoothly and in order to ensure a safe introduction of this policy supervisors are currently notified of all midwife bookings. A continuous audit of outcomes ensures that amendment to the guidelines can be readily published and new (colour coded) copies circulated to all midwives. Involving midwives in the development of policies has provided midwives with ownership and the ability to answer criticism more constructively when things don't go smoothly.

Supervision and midwives

Supervision and choice

Historically at Southmead, supervision and manager roles have been embodied in one person and this may have predisposed to some confusion on the part of midwives regarding the role of the supervisor. Any failure in the interpersonal relationships within this arrangement means that the midwife could lack both managerial and supervisory support. The team discussed this issue and to resolve any potential difficulties decided to offer midwives a choice of supervisor and the opportunity to change supervisor with ease if they wish.

As an introduction to this new system (and fearing administrative chaos) each midwife was allocated a named supervisor but was also given the option of changing supervisor. A number of midwives chose to change supervisor having gained information of the supervisor's interests and expertise (via the booklet mentioned earlier) as well as personal preference based on other knowledge. The scheme is being further developed in this 'supervisory year', with more information about supervision being made available to midwives, and a completely free choice of named supervisor on a first reply basis until the supervisor's caseload is full. Each supervisor also selects a named supervisor from the team to supervise their practise.

Access

A key factor in the effectiveness of supervision is the accessibility of the supervisor to midwives, both in theory and in practice. Although midwives had access to a supervisor of midwives (on a 24 hour basis) this was previously only achieved via the midwife managing the maternity unit at the time. To improve access, the pager number was made available to all midwives. A small 'credit card' sized business card, which can be stored unobtrusively in a wallet containing details of how to contact the supervisor is currently being piloted. This will ensure that all midwives could have the pager number readily available.

Having attempted to address the practical aspects of access, attention was focused on to whether the midwife *actually* contacts a supervisor for advice on professional issues. An audit was undertaken to identify the reasons why supervisors were contacted. Other occasions subsequently came to the supervisors' attention indicating that despite the midwife either requiring advice or with hindsight recognized that supervisory advice would still be beneficial, a supervisor was *not* contacted. The supervisory team is concerned to investigate the reasons for this. This information is obviously difficult to obtain but has the potential to demonstrate midwives real access to supervisory support. Some midwives continue to appear reluctant to contact the supervisor regarding professional issues but confident to phone over non professional issues (e.g. a problem with the heating system). One possibility is that midwives do not understand the role of the supervisor and more information about the supervisors role is being included in this year's 'supervisors' booklet'.

Weekly multidisciplinary audit meetings to discuss the care provided to individual women (in an anonymous manner) have been arranged. As Southmead is a large unit, anonymity is often possible, particularly as examples of good, bad and questionable care management or practice are all discussed rather than the meeting focusing on 'incidents'. Midwives and medical staff are invited to discuss care they were involved with, particularly if it was unusual (e.g. puerperal psychosis), or details of a care plan for a woman not yet delivered which is in some way complicated. Aspects of the supervisors' role can be raised at this meeting and included in the discussion further raising the profile of midwifery supervision. Increasing midwives' true accessibility to the supervisor remains a complex issue which supervisors are attempting to address in various ways, including building relationships. Some midwives have not accepted the invitation to attend a supervisory interview this year and there is some dilemma about how to react to this. If midwives are offered an interview and decline the temptation is to coerce attendance in the interests of meeting the supervision quality standards. The introduction of more clinically based supervisors may improve access to supervision for some midwives.

Providing support to midwives

The first step to providing midwives with support is obviously to ensure access to the supervisor as has already been described. The following are, in my experience, broad areas in which the midwife may require support:

- Practice development.

- Support to provide care that a woman requests (particularly when the midwife considers the care inappropriate).

- Investigating allegations of poor practice.

- Recognizing poor practice related to health issues.

- Support in the event of litigation.

These situations are obviously very diverse and rather than suggest solutions to various hypothetical problems, a description of the tools which the supervisory team has found helpful might aid supervisors in other situations. Confidentiality is vitally important in the supervisory relationship and this must be respected as far as possible. Depending on the circumstances however, the supervisor may be better able to offer advice to the midwife if the issue is brought to the attention of the supervisory team (in an anonymous manner if possible). This will provide the supervisor with support, as well as enabling 'supervision' of the supervisor. In such situations confidentiality within the supervisory team is paramount.

Women should, in the future, be better informed about maternity care and be more empowered to make decisions about their pregnancy. This needs to be encouraged, and facilitated by the provision of research based literature to all women. Some women will still decide to request inappropriate care. Other women may request care that research indicates is satisfactory but the prejudice of health professionals and a lack of research based practice places the woman in a situation of having to defend her request. The professional groups involved i.e. midwife, general practitioner, obstetrician and paediatrician may all have different views on the care that is most appropriate. The woman may rapidly find herself in the unenviable position of having inadequate support and feeling totally disempowered.

Women may at this point contact the supervisor of midwives or the service manager (who may be the same person). Without wishing to diminish or detract from the primary relationship that the midwife has with the women, a meeting with the woman, her partner and midwife should be offered. This early 'fact finding' meeting will enable the supervisor to discover what the woman is actually requesting and enable the supervisor to be an informed advocate for the mother and baby (ENB, 1994). The supervisor can support the midwife in obtaining the most recent valid research and in discussing the request with other professionals involved. This is particularly helpful when the midwife is facing criticism from other professionals for providing care which is a legal responsibility, irrespective of the circumstances. The active involvement of the supervisor (irrespective of any contact with the woman) will support the midwife through what can be a very stressful time.

The supervisor, who is also the manager, is in a very complex position as the manager has a different range of responsibilities within the employee/employer relationship. The manger may be required by the Trust to contact the woman to discuss her request for a type of care which is not within the service specification of the Trust. A supervisor in such a situation must be overtly aware of which 'hat' she is wearing.

Investigating allegations of poor practice

Allegations of poor practice may become evident through a clinical incident, internal audit (e.g. records), reports by midwives, doctors, women or their families and on direct observation by the supervisor. The supervisor must investigate the allegation and decide how the issues are to be addressed. In some circumstances an employment disciplinary procedure will also be instigated. Depending on the circumstances, the supervisor may choose to undertake the investigation herself, or request that a colleague investigate the issue. The supervisor must come to a judgement as to whether the incident should be reported to the Local Supervising Authority (LSA). Whatever the process or outcome, it is important that the midwife has access to a named supervisor who is independent of the investigation and can provide support. If allegations of poor practice are made it is essential that the midwife is given written information about the allegation and the opportunity to respond. Records should be maintained of all supervisory discussions, and copies given to the midwife. If appropriate, a programme of updating and supervised practice should be arranged. The advice of a midwifery tutor should be obtained when formulating aims and objectives for midwives to ensure the methodology is sound. Short or long term ill health may be the cause of poor practice and this should be taken into account by the supervisor. Expert advice is available via occupational health physicians.

Poor practice can also be a 'cultural' issue involving a large number of midwives. A different approach is beneficial in resolving such practice issues, involving the utilization of audit information, detailed analysis of the issues and the development of a strategy to improve practice as discussed earlier.

Litigation

Litigation in maternity services may become more common and my personal experience is that midwives can be very poor at making statements and become anxious at the prolonged legal process. A named supervisor within the supervisory team who has developed an interest and additional knowledge about the process of litigation who can advise and support midwives at such times is an advantage. An arrangement exists at Southmead to ensure that supervisors are involved appropriately with any litigation process and the midwife is offered support from a supervisor when making statements to the solicitor.

Supervisory records

Supervisors are required to maintain records of all supervisory activities. The form of these records is not defined by the English National Board, but presumably could be defined by the LSA. Such records should include details of supervisory reviews, a copy of which should be retained by the midwife. It can be beneficial to the midwife if the supervisory record and any self preparation or self assessment are in a format which is suitable for inclusion in the midwife's personal portfolio. An example of such a supervisory review form is given is the 'Preparation of Supervisors of Midwives' pack (ENB, 1992). Experimenting with different types of documentation each year has led to greater thought about the annual review process by the supervisory team and gives fresh stimulus to the approach.

Supervisory review must not be confused with employment appraisal, but if the midwife selects a supervisor who is also her manager there are obviously areas of overlap. Supervisors should consider how they will approach this area of overlap to avoid duplication. A system which has been helpful at Southmead has been to ensure that the supervisory and appraisal documentation are complimentary enabling the discussions to be of a complementary nature.

Supervision and women

Supervision of midwifery has a long history, but little is known about the role outside of the profession (and arguably misunderstood within the profession). Supervisors can be instrumental in facilitating choice for women. Supervisors may wish to address the issue of how women access their support within the local area and this can be achieved by using whatever resources are already available. For example, including a brief description of the function of the supervisor in any information booklets which are produced including details of the role of the supervisor in supporting women's choice. Contact information should obviously be included. Supervisors could arrange to meet with volunteers involved with local support groups e.g. National Childbirth Trust (NCT), Stillbirth and Neonatal Death Society (SANDS), Miscarriage Association. If a working relationship is formed with counsellors working within such lay organizations, general feedback on the midwifery service can be obtained and issues resolved. Some women approach the Community Health Council (CHC), particularly if they have a complaint or require information. Good relationships between the supervisor and the CHC representative will facilitate faster and easier communication for these women.

Supervision and audit

Within the economic and political climate in which midwives now practice, it is imperative that the effectiveness of supervision is measured. Audit of the standard of midwifery supervision is becoming more common with annual reports of the activities of supervisors being required by the LSA. Supervision should however be an integral part of midwifery practice and service provision. Consequently auditing changes and improvements in maternity care that are purely attributable to midwifery supervision is unlikely to be possible. A more helpful and realistic approach may be to audit the ways in which midwifery supervision has influenced midwifery practice, the development of maternity services and the care offered to women.

Development	Role of Midwifery Supervision
Improvement in the rate of women breastfeeding at 6 weeks postnatal.	Audit of existing rates Compilation of new breastfeeding guidelines by multidisciplinary group. Midwives knowledge and attitudes to breastfeeding discussed at supervisory reviews. Breastfeeding workshops held by supervisor for health care assistants
Implementation of two additional community based teams.	Audit of experience of midwives planning to join the team. Development of individual updating programmes for midwives joining the teams. Home birth work shops Negociation of service change with GPs

Fig.7.4: Role of midwifery supervision in the development of maternity services

The influence of supervisory activities should be included in the annual report, written in a style and format which is attractive to a wide audience e.g. midwives, managers and lay organizations.

Conclusion

Within a rapidly changing health care environment, it is essential that midwifery supervision continues to move away from professional isolation focused solely on an introspective interest in midwifery, to appreciating wider political and social agendas. There have, of course, always been courageous midwives who have campaigned for the rights of women in childbirth. Supervisors could take a fuller role in this arena in the future and may be forced to do so if 'Changing Childbirth' (Department of Health, 1993) is to be fully implemented. Greater political awareness of current health issues and health trends will enable supervisors to both learn from and contribute to wider health debates thus raising the profile of the profession. Supervisors should consider the current national and local health care issues and consider midwifery services and care against that backdrop. The model of professional supervision experienced by midwives is unique and that uniqueness may lead to misunderstanding by others. When considering midwifery supervision it is imperative that good practice includes good communication with other professional teams, as well as concentrating on the issues which relate directly to midwifery practice.

References

Belbin, R. (1981). *Management Teams: Why They Succeed or Fail*. London: Butterworth-Heinemann.

Department of Health (1993). *Report of the Expert Advisory Group: Changing Childbirth*. London: HMSO.

ENB (1992). *Preparation of Supervisors of Midwives*. London: ENB.

ENB (1994). *Supervision of Midwives*. London: ENB.

Johnson, G., Scholes, K. (1993). *Exploring Corporate Strategy*. Cambridge: Prentice Hall.

Kakabadse, A., Ludlow, R., Vinnicombe, S. (1988). *Working in Organizations*. Harmondsworth: Penguin.

Kolb, D.A. (1984). *Experiential Learning*. London: Prentice Hall.

Mintzberg, H. (1973). *The Nature of Managerial Work*. New York: London: Harper & Row.

Mintzberg, H., Quinn, J.B. (1991). *The Strategy Process: Concepts, Contexts, Cases*. Second Edition. Englewood Cliffs, NJ: Prentice Hall.

Mottram, R. (1982). 'Team skills management'. *Journal of Management Development*. Vol 1., No.1 pp.22-33.

Schon, E. (1990). *Educating the Reflective Practitioner*. San Francisco: Jossey Bass.

Stewart, R. (1982). *Choices for the Manager: A Guide to Managerial Work*. New York: Mcgraw-Hill.

UKCC (1994). *The Midwives Code of Practice*. London: UKCC.

CHAPTER EIGHT

Supervision and Practice Change at King's

> **Cathy Warwick RGN, RM, MSc (Sociology), BSc (Nursing), PGCEA, ADM**
> is currently General Manager of Women's and Children's Services/Director of Midwifery and Gynaecology at King's Healthcare NHS Trust in South East London. She has also worked in education, both as a midwife teacher at St Mary's Hospital, Paddington and Director of Midwifery in the North London College of Health Studies. She is particulary interested in women becoming more involved in the planning and development of maternity services.

The publication of the Cumberlege Report (Department of Health, 1993) and its subsequent acceptance as Government policy in August 1993 created the potential and impetus for change in the maternity services. The report states clearly that maternity services should be women centred and that women want choice, continuity and control throughout their antenatal, labour and postnatal care. Furthermore the report emphasizes the need for services to be accessible to all women.

The report has major implications for obstetricians, general practitioners and midwives. In order to ensure that the aims of the report are fulfilled, it is essential not only that the best possible use is made of the different but complimentary skills of these three groups but also that they work together to achieve a co-ordinated approach to practice change.

King's Healthcare NHS Trust is a large teaching hospital in South East London. Maternity services are provided to approximately 3700 women a year. The inner city catchment area typically creates a multi ethnic population with a high level of social deprivation (LSL, 1995).

There is support at King's for practice change in line with the recommendations of the Cumberlege Report (Department of Health, 1993). For a variety of reasons however the approach has been one of gradual evolution as opposed to sudden and comprehensive change. This is felt to be appropriate because:

- staff have already experienced major changes in recent years including the amalgamation of two maternity units and the alteration of established working patterns.

- it is not yet clear what model of practice is ideal for meeting the report's recommendations and it is important to evaluate both new models and current models (Walsh, 1995).

- some midwives require further continuing education before they are ready to meet the report's recommendations.

- midwives are at different points of readiness to adopt changes in working patterns.

- there is evidence in consumer surveys of satisfaction on the part of some women with particular models of care even if these don't enable continuity of care in labour (Lee, 1994).

An evolutionary approach ensures:

- that staff are not overwhelmed by too rapid and too much change.
- that changes can be evaluated and models adapted to meet particular needs both of the women and of aspects of the service.
- that the impact of new models of care on staff can be reviewed and models adapted so that they are acceptable to staff thus enhancing the likelihood of the success of that model.
- that current practice which is of a good standard is not sacrificed for the sake of new models of care which are not yet evaluated.
- that programmes of education can prepare midwives for practice change.

The development of midwifery practices

Since August 1993 the focus of change at King's has been the development of midwifery practices. Each practice has emerged from an idea originally put forward by either an individual midwife, a group of midwives or a group of midwives and general practitioners (GPs). One by one these practices have been established until in November 1995, seven practices have the potential to provide care to 1200 women.

The practice model of care currently runs in tandem with a 'traditional' model of care. The latter model of care describes a system where a woman usually meets different care givers in the antenatal, labour and postnatal period. This fragmentation of care will be most evident in women having full hospital care and less evident in women who receive care from the same community staff antenatally and postnatally. In some aspects of the 'traditional' system i.e. community midwifery, homebirths and domino schemes continuity of care is high and women entering these schemes will receive a model of care which is similar to women who become part of a practice caseload. Through audit and evaluation of the two models further change will emerge.

Practices are staffed by four to six midwives and have a defined caseload of 40 bookings per midwife per year. Care is provided in the community and the hospital throughout the antenatal, labour and postnatal periods. The practice midwives attend between 80 per cent and 90 per cent of their births. Births take place at home as well as in hospital.

The model reflects the findings of Wraight et al (1993) that if teams of midwives are to achieve the aim of providing continuity of care, there is most chance of doing so if the following features apply:

- the team consists of no more than six midwives
- each team has a defined caseload
- the team provides total care for that caseload
- the team works in all areas according to client need
- fifty percent or more of women are delivered by a midwife known to her.

Apart from these general principles, all the practices are slightly different because they vary in the way they select their caseloads. Four practices have a caseload based on the total population of women registering with a GP practice. Depending on the location of the GP practice, this will create differing caseloads in terms of social deprivation and ethnic mix with ensuing variation in needs.

Three practices base their caseload on women with particular needs e.g. young unsupported women, women with previous pregnancy loss and women with a history of mental illness. In addition one of these practices offers a homebirth service to women who are not supported in this request by their GP.

Although efforts have been made nationally to categorize a group of women who are at low risk and who are therefore suitable for antenatal care and delivery outside a consultant led obstetric unit (Cole, 1994; Bull, 1994), the practices at King's offer care to women regardless of their status as high or low risk, whether this is defined at the onset of pregnancy or during the antenatal period. This is possible because the practice midwives offer care in community and hospital settings, work in a compact geographical area and liaise closely with a named obstetrician.

Direct access to a consultant obstetrician or consultant paediatrician at any time for advice and support is considered to be important. This is not just because the practices are looking after low and high risk women. The 'Report on Confidential Enquiries into Maternal Deaths in the United Kingdom 1988-90' (Department of Health, 1994 p.163) identified that 'in a significant number of cases there is clear evidence of lack of availability of appropriate staff to deal with major problems'. The 'Report of the Confidential Enquiry into Stillbirths and Deaths in Infancy' (Department of Health, 1995) also highlighted a range of communication issues including that of poor relationships between professionals. It is hoped that the establishment of clear links between practice midwives and an appropriate level of obstetric and paediatric staff can overcome many difficulties and reduce risk. Kitzinger et al. (Garcia, 1990) discuss the benefits that can result from a staffing structure that involves midwives and consultants working more closely together including appropriate consultant supervision for women, increased confidence in midwives to discuss issues, an increasingly two way process of communication resulting in more respect of midwives by consultants and the ensuing potential for developing a more autonomous and powerful midwifery role.

For the majority of women booking into their caseload a midwife will be the lead professional defined in the 'Cumberlege Report' (Department of Health, 1993) as the person who has a key role in the planning and provision of her care. In addition the midwives as a practice must set and monitor their standards of organization and care and determine their own working patterns and arrangements for off duty and on call. The midwives cover their own sickness and study leave.

A philosophy of support

The effect of working in a practice is that midwives are more clearly accountable for the work that they do and the standard of clinical care they provide than has usually been the case when working in systems which offer less continuity of care.

A few midwives will adapt very readily to practice work but for the majority of midwives, and indeed obstetricians and general practitioners, establishing this model of care presents many challenges and good quality support is vital. In the later stages of development the challenges will be different but effective supervision will still be crucial to the successful working of a small team.

Support is required in relation to four key areas:

- adaptation to a new model of working
- education and training
- setting and auditing clinical standards
- establishing and maintaining effective inter professional relationships.

The system must also ensure that those who interrelate with the practices receive support, otherwise conflicts both interprofessionally and among midwives may undermine the model of care. Women must also be helped to understand different models of care.

The philosophy at King's is that, if this new model of care is to be successful and women ultimately to benefit, the supervision of midwives must be conducted in a way which enables midwives to grow and develop. The climate must be one which encourages openness and honesty and which engenders a sense of trust. Innovation must be encouraged. Reflection both on practice and on working patterns should be fostered as should a sense of learning together. Hierarchical structures may remain but with the purpose of providing support rather than control.

There must also be clarity about how support is to be provided. It cannot simply be given in an ad hoc way as this inevitably means that it only comes into play when problems arise. Ongoing, formal support ensures a proactive approach which anticipates challenges and ensures that when problems do arise there is a cohesive group which can come together to resolve them.

The mechanisms of support

The key aspect of providing effective support has been to set up mechanisms for regular, structured meetings with each of the midwifery practices.

Each practice meets with the lead supervisor, who is also the Director of Midwifery, once a month. Other managers and supervisors may attend the meeting but if they are unable to do so they will receive minutes and issues which affect them will be addressed with them by the Director of Midwifery.

These meetings:

- provide a forum at which advice can be given on day to day issues
- allow reflection on a new system of care provision and continued adaptation of that system
- ensure a formal record of practice evolution is available to inform future practice development
- help new practices to learn from the experiences of established practices.

Three key areas are discussed:

- What is needed in order to support the midwives in their work? Have they got adequate equipment and communication systems, is secretarial support available?
- Are they achieving the agreed contract of care? This will involve both quantitative and qualitative data e.g. what are their booking and delivery numbers, how many of the births of their women have they been able to attend, what are their breastfeeding rates?
- Women under their care: e.g. are there any particular difficulties with which they need support or help, have they undertaken any deliveries on which they would like to reflect?

The meetings are minuted.

In addition every three months a joint meeting is held between midwifery supervisors and all of the group practices.

In recognition of the fact that the new model of care has an impact on the more 'traditional' model further monthly meetings are held between:

- the labour ward midwives
- the community midwives (each of the three areas has a separate meeting)
- other hospital midwives.

At these meetings, among other issues, the impact of the existence of midwifery practices on the work of core staff is discussed. For example, the midwife in charge of the labour ward was unclear of her own relationship to a practice midwife attending a woman in labour. An open discussion ensured clarification of a midwife's accountability for the clinical care of a woman, of the potential nonetheless for support of a less experienced midwife from a more experienced midwife and of the importance of good communication between practice midwives and the person who must ensure the smooth running of a busy environment.

Finally meetings are held with GPs, obstetricians and consumer groups to ensure that inter professional relationships are clear, that patterns of working are well established and that there is a clear understanding of what is being offered to women. These meetings take place on an 'as required' basis.

As noted earlier, establishing appropriate obstetric links is particularly important. Midwives who are taking responsibility for a woman's care are not properly respected in that role if, when they refer for advice, they find themselves in consultation with a junior doctor who has less experience than themselves. At King's obstetric and paediatric staff have been happy to ensure that midwives have access to a senior registrar or a consultant. There is a designated consultant linked to each midwifery practice.

GPs have been concerned that developments in midwifery practice will undermine their own role in maternity care. It has been important for midwifery supervisors to spend time with individual GP practices discussing the form of midwifery input that would be most valuable to themselves and explaining the different types of developments happening within the area they work. Considerable time has also been spent at GP forums and written information has been printed in GP newsletters.

All practice changes are discussed at the Maternity Service Liaison Committee. This is attended by four consumer representatives from:

- the National Childbirth Trust (NCT)
- the Community Health Council (CHC)
- the Black and Ethnic Minorities Health Action Group (BEMHAG)
- the Disabilities Action Group.

In addition, time has been spent attending consumer forums, NCT teachers' groups and NCT local meetings.

The main aim in relating closely with consumer groups is to find out how they wish to see practice developing. A second aim is to ensure that they understand the constraints on the pace of change and the rationale behind the evolutionary approach. In addition it is helpful for them to understand the degree of continuity that is possible. All this ensures that women have realistic expectations of the service midwives can offer.

A flavour of what is happening

Adaptation to new patterns of working
When midwives join a midwifery practice they radically change their working patterns. Shifts, regular rotation between day and night duty and chunks of time spent in any one clinical area are features of the 'traditional' model of care. Midwives will experience a new challenge of on call work and rapid change not only from one area of care to another but also between hospital and community.

The peaks and troughs inevitable in any maternity service will not just mean a busy shift, but possibly a busy three or four days often followed by a guilt-inducing quiet spell. The anxiety of being on call even if a midwife is not actually called may affect sleep patterns and a normal social life.

Midwives have welcomed the opportunity to talk about the impact of this change. Through discussion, adjustment has been made to working patterns and to the numbers of midwives in the practices to ensure pressure of on call work does not decrease motivation and result in burn out.

It is important to emphasize, however, that decisions about change always come from the midwives themselves and the role of the supervisor is to facilitate discussion and introduce ideas, not to impose solutions.

For example, it was the view of midwifery supervisors that one particular practice, which delivers 50 per cent of its women at home, needed to increase the number of midwives working within it. This practice only had three midwives and due to their decision to provide a first and second on call midwife they were effectively on call two nights out of three.

The practice were convinced that it would destroy their philosophy of care if they increased their numbers and various other solutions were explored e.g. linking with another practice to cover the second on call or altering their caseload to create a different balance between home and hospital births or indeed reconsideration of whether a second on call was necessary.

For a month or so the practice considered these solutions and ultimately requested the allocation of an additional midwife to the practice. This was a major change and it was vital that it was a decision owned by themselves.

More than ever before, midwives need to be good team workers. During the course of monthly meetings practice members are encouraged to establish their agreed ground rules. Experience has shown how important it is that everyone knows what is and can be expected of each other and that the established norms are made clear to women.

One practice faced a particular problem when on two occasions women requested not be to be attended by one member of their group. The practice had to decide whether this was a possible option or not for these particular women and whether it would be possible in future. They also had to address what was behind this request. On a later occasion having had a male midwife join the practice, they had to decide whether the principle they had decided upon - which was to encourage women not to see it as an option to choose among members - still applied. Once again the purpose of the supervision meetings was not to make these decisions but to ensure that among themselves the midwives found a solution.

New working patterns require different and appropriate communication systems and equipment. Monthly meetings have been invaluable in discussing the infrastructure that is required to support each practice. Although the provision of new equipment creates additional expense it became clear at monthly meetings that stress among midwives was often related to this being inadequate. It also created the potential for women delivering unaided if one set of central equipment had to be collected prior to attending a homebirth. Mobile phones, message pagers and BT charge cards are now part of practice equipment. Booking in the community requires midwives to be equipped with lap top computers and an increasing number of home births mean all midwives will require a set of neonatal resuscitation equipment.

Education and training

Practice meetings establish a forum at which the midwives can discuss emerging clinical issues and the type of educational needs associated with them. Midwives require education and training support to alter their work patterns. At King's four issues have been identified as being of crucial importance (Warwick, 1995):

- Firstly, if midwives are to be able to empower women they themselves must be empowered. They must be helped to understand themselves and have knowledge of their own strengths, weaknesses and prejudices. Such insight is fundamental to attitude change and a move from relationships with women based on professional power to ones based on partnership is necessary.

- Secondly, midwives require help to develop skills of decision making within an analytical framework. Concepts of risk and choice involve placing facts in a total clinical context that include the feelings of the woman, her family and indeed the staff caring for her.

An excellent knowledge of facts and an ability to access information are not in themselves adequate. The context in which they are placed may result in many possible outcomes and options for care, all of which may be equally valid.

Making decisions within an analytical framework requires the midwife to understand the culture, values and expectations of the woman, her family, the professionals involved and perhaps the wider public.

- Thirdly, midwives must feel confident of having the necessary skills and knowledge to provide flexible, women centred care. Working in group practices they must be able to provide the full range of care whether in the home or hospital setting. Training in the following areas has been of particular importance:

  - Information Technology (IT) skills enabling midwives to carry out computerized home bookings
  - Neonatal resuscitation and intravenous cannulation to ensure safety at home confinements
  - Perineal suturing to allow continuity of care in labour.

- Midwives must know how to access knowledge and how to interpret information. Education in information retrieval and research awareness is extremely important.

The pressure to achieve major change within existing resources is high and in many maternity units, training and development of midwives is seen as a luxury. This is surely regrettable. Unless the educational development of midwives mirrors and enhances service development, the possibility of achieving real change is unlikely.

A variety of education opportunities have been developed addressing all of these issues and midwives are released to attend courses, study days and workshops (currently of the 33 practice midwives nine are studying for a degree in midwifery). Workshops have been set up on specific factual topics. For example, concern was expressed about inadequate knowledge of antenatal screening tests for fetal abnormality. This has resulted in the provision of a series of half day workshops which all midwives providing antenatal care will attend.

Midwives working in one practice where part of their caseload is referred by a group of psychiatrists were discussing the strain that a very needy group of women was placing on them. They now have regular clinical supervision sessions with a nurse teacher who is also a trained mental nurse. This helps them to understand more fully the needs of the women in their caseload with mental health problems.

Apprenticeship learning is also encouraged. Many midwives are enthusiastic and highly motivated but they may need time working with experienced midwives before they feel confident in a setting which requires more autonomy and sometimes very different skills. Supervisors must be prepared to give them the time to develop at their own pace. At King's the decision as to whether or not a midwife is ready to undertake homebirths on her own responsibility is determined through self and peer appraisal. A climate of support has resulted in a service where 40 per cent of the midwives are now able to provide this service.

Clinical standards and audit

Very general standards can be drawn from the Cumberlege Report (Department of Health, 1993) and from various other policy documents relating to the maternity services. These as well as standards relating to the Patient's Charter and to service specifications agreed with purchasers will apply to the midwifery practices as well as to the whole maternity service.

As a new model of care, midwifery practices are encouraged both to set additional standards and to monitor specific aspects of their practice. For example, some concern has been expressed by local GPs that practice midwives may achieve continuity in labour at the expense of continuity in the antenatal period as midwives try to ensure that women in the practice know all the midwives. At the monthly meetings, discussion takes place as to how this aspect of practice will be audited and the practices are encouraged to decide what an acceptable number of different contacts is in the antenatal period.

Standards also become very important as women's expectations of the services increase and resources remain finite. Midwives must be prepared to sit down and work out clearly what they can offer with the resources available. For example:

- what is the normal length of a booking visit at home?
- can all women expect to be assessed at home in early labour?
- will practice midwives undertake to do the postnatal care of their women when they are in hospital or are the core staff expected to cover?

Clarity in these areas is important for women but also ensures that there is good communication with midwifery colleagues who are still working within the more 'traditional' pattern of care.

Audit is becoming much more a reality of daily life for midwives working in practices. They are directly involved in the collection of information and the results of audit are discussed at the monthly meetings. Midwives are becoming increasingly interested in the outcomes for their caseload e.g. caesarean section rates, breastfeeding rates and in comparing these outcomes against other models of care and analysing the reason for differences.

Inter-professional relationships

Each practice development has been based on an idea proposed by midwives working in clinical settings. Often ideas have been developed in co-operation with the GPs with whom midwives have been working. Building on the ideas of practitioners and enabling midwives and GPs to participate together from the very beginning in developments has ensured a high level of ownership and commitment as well as co-operative working. Inter-professional rivalry has been minimized and mutual respect has flourished.

It has been important that the consultants with whom midwives link have a positive view of midwifery practice developments and are sympathetic towards the ideal of women centred care. They too must be prepared to work co-operatively with midwives and to enable women to make choices based on research based advice and information. Obstetricians who may have had a less positive outlook on developments have been impressed at such co-operative working and have tended to develop an increasing interest in such models of care.

It is through reflection on cases that most is learned about inter-professional working. The monthly meeting with supervisors not only allows midwives to reflect on midwifery practice but gives supervisors the opportunity to suggest situations in which discussion with relevant other professionals may be appropriate. It also allows midwifery supervisors to identify when other professionals are not adopting an individualised approach to care and to discuss with colleagues how this might be rectified.

Conclusion

The style of supervision can affect whether or not midwives will be able to change their practice in a way which ensures that the wishes of women are met. Emphasis must be on support and counselling. Midwives need to be helped and encouraged to take on new roles and responsibilities. If aspects of their work are less than satisfactory they will learn most through reflection and discussion in an atmosphere of trust.

Supervision of course primarily exists to protect women and their babies and there will always be extreme cases when a disciplinary approach is warranted. Normally however high standards will emerge more effectively if midwives are treated themselves as they are expected to treat women. Midwives must be empowered themselves before they can empower women.

Case discussion with an emphasis on effective care and audit are vital elements of a system which aims to increase the midwives insight into her daily practice.

Change is not a process that can happen overnight. The pace of change that is possible will depend on many issues including that of resources. Most crucially it will depend on the ability of the midwives to embrace new models of care. The model must be one which is both achievable by the current workforce and fulfils the expectations of the women. If these two are to be compatible it is dependent to a large extent on the supervisor of midwives having a regular dialogue both with midwives and with women to discuss what can be expected and achieved.

Midwifery practices allow effective small group supervision. This does not detract from the need for individual supervision and it is important that the needs of individuals are not submerged in the needs of the group.

It is clear that certain management styles create a process which is very similar to good supervision. However in the new models of care developed at King's, midwives are not so closely managed and supervision of midwives becomes increasingly important. The monthly meetings described ensure an established focus for communication and feedback.

References

Bull, M. (1994). 'Selection of women for community obstetric care' in Chamberlain, G., Patel, N. (Eds). *The Future of the Maternity Services*. pp.73-81. London: RCOG Press.

Cole, S., McIlwaine, G. (1994). 'The use of risk factors in predicting possible consequences of changing patterns of care in pregnancy' in Chamberlain, G., Patel, N. (Eds). *The Future of the Maternity Services*, pp.73-81. London: RCOG Press.

Department of Health (1993). *Changing Childbirth Report of the Expert Maternity Group* (The Cumberlege Report). HMSO: London.

Department of Health (1994). *Report on Confidential Enquiries into Maternal Deaths in the United Kingdom 1988-1990*. London: HMSO.

Department of Health (1995). *Confidential Enquiry into Stillbirths and Deaths in Infancy*. Part 1 - summary of methods and main results. London: HMSO.

Kitzinger, J. et al. (1990). 'Labour relations: midwives and doctors on the labour ward' in Garcia, Jo et al. (Eds). *The Politics of Maternity Care*, pp.149-162. Oxford: Oxford University Press.

Lambeth, Southwark and Lewisham Health Commission (1995). *The Future of Primary Health Care in South East London.* 1 Lower Marsh, London SE1.

Lee, G. (1994). 'A reassuring familiar face?' *Nursing Times* 90, (17), pp.66-67.

Walsh, D. (1995). 'Continuity of carer: miracle or mirage?' *British Journal of Midwifery*, Vol. 3, No. 6, pp.336-338.

Warwick, C., Jamieson, L (1995). 'Educating for change in midwifery services' *Professional Update*, Vol. 3, No. 8, Pearson Professional Ltd.

Wraight, A. et al. (1993). *Mapping Team Midwifery*: a report to the Department of Health. Brighton: Institute of Manpower Studies.

CHAPTER NINE

Audit of Supervisors in the West Midlands

Ann Skipworth RGN, RM, ADM
is the Directorate Manager (Obstetrics, Gynaecology and Paedriatrics) with the Dudley Group of Hospitals, NHS Trust, West Midlands, combining the role of Business Manager and Professional Head of Services. Prior to this role she has been Director of Nursing and Midwifery at Birmingham Maternity Hospital, and is Link Supervisor for the West Midlands.

Background

During the 1980s the profile of supervisors and supervision of midwifery practice in the West Midlands was continuously being raised, with initiatives planned and implemented by a small group of experienced supervisors, supported and encouraged by the Regional Nursing Officer (RNO).

In 1989 it was recognized that although supervisors carried out their role with guidance from the United Kingdom Central Council for Nursing, Midwifery and Health Visiting (UKCC) and English National Board (ENB), there were no local standards for supervisors. There was concern that there were a small number of supervisors who did not fully understand their role and therefore concern that their performance may not have been of the expected standard.

The small working group undertook responsibility for formulating ten standards for supervisors with the design based on the now well used DySSSy (Dynamic Standard Setting System - Royal College of Nursing, 1990) with each standard containing a main statement, followed by details of the structure, process and outcome facilitating those using the standards to implement them. The draft was circulated to the co-ordinating supervisors in the region for comment, amendments were made where appropriate and the final document circulated to all supervisors in 1991. The standards included are set out below:

1. Each supervisor of midwives has a clear understanding of the statutory responsibilities.
2. Each practising midwife is personally aware of her named supervisor of midwives, and other supervisors within the district.
3. The supervisor of midwives ensures that each practising midwife maintains her knowledge and skills at a level required by the UKCC.

4. The supervisor of midwives ensures that Rule 36 in the Handbook of Midwives Rules and section 3.1 of A Midwife's Code of Practice are complied with by each midwife within her area of responsibility.
5. The supervisor of midwives ensures each midwife is competent to practise skills.
6. The supervisor of midwives ensures that Rule 41 in the Handbook of Midwives Rules and section 3.4 of A Midwife's Code of Practice are complied with by each midwife within her area of responsibility.
7. The supervisor of midwives ensures that Rule 42 in the Handbook of Midwives Rules and section 3.5 of A Midwife's Code of Practice are complied with by each midwife within her area of responsibility.
8. The supervisor of midwives ensures that Rule 37 in the Handbook of Midwives Rules and section 3.2 of A Midwife's Code of Practice are complied with by each midwife within her area of responsibility.
9. The supervisor of midwives investigates and takes action when allegations are made of misconduct or unacceptable midwifery practice.
10. The supervisor of midwives provides support and advice to midwives undertaking home confinements within her area of responsibility, to ensure the best possible care is provided for the mother and her baby.

At that point there had been no consideration of taking this work further.

Audit

During the next few months, it was evident from discussion with the supervisors that the standards were proving useful to them and enabling them to undertake their role in a more structured manner. However, during the following 18 month period it was recognized that if one considered the quality cycle (see Fig 9.1), we had only completed

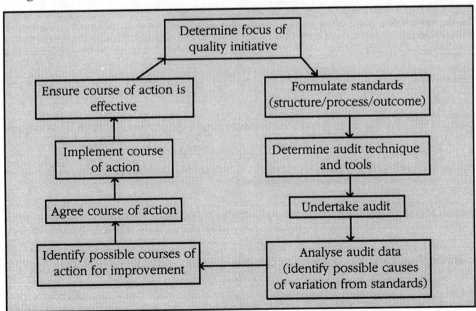

Fig. 9.1: The Quality Cycle (amended from Ellis, R., Whittington, D 1993 *Quality Assurance in Health Care*, London: Edward Arnold.)

a small part of the circle. The next essential step was to undertake audits in order for the performance of supervisors to be checked against the standards we had set.

Audit has been defined in several ways.

Chambers Dictionary (1980) states the following:

> 'The examination of accounts by an authorized person or persons; a calling to account generally; a statement of account; a periodic settlement of accounts'.

whilst the Concise Oxford Dictionary (1988) gives a briefer definition:

> 'Official examination of accounts'.

It is accepted that the idea of audit is a common element in quality assurance, with Ellis and Whittington (1993) describing quality audit as 'an audit of an organization's quality assurance procedures to ascertain whether they are operating as stated and meeting their objectives'. They continue to explain that 'audit is sometimes used in a broader sense to cover any checking of reality against stated or predicted standards'.

It therefore became essential for an audit tool to be designed and a system of audit agreed.

Within the region, which at that time contained 22 District Health Authorities, there were between 80 - 100 supervisors at any given time and therefore, the most important areas for consideration were:

- How would the audit be conducted?
- By whom?
- When?
- How?

By whom

Three possibilities were discussed:

- Audit by the Local Supervising Authority (LSA) officer
- Peer group audit in each district
- Audit supervisors from another district.

Although the LSA Officer made annual visits to all districts, these meetings were on a 'group' basis. It was agreed that the requirement for audit of individual supervisors - on a 'one-to-one' basis - would be difficult for her to achieve because of the large number of supervisors. Peer group audit is widely accepted, (Royal College of General Practitioners, 1983) and could be used by supervisors, as there is supposedly no hierarchical structure in supervision. However this option was discounted for two reasons.

Firstly the non-hierarchical framework is often ignored by supervisors who hold managerial positions above the level of their colleagues. Secondly, from previous experience it is sometimes difficult for a supervisor to make constructive critical comments on a colleague's performance, especially if the critic has less experience of supervision.

Neither of the reasons should be accepted but we know that these situations can be found in many areas. Having now ruled out two of the options, the third was debated at length and eventual agreement reached that this would be the way forward in our region. We were not aware of any other region who had adopted this approach and realized that we were moving into 'uncharted waters'.

It was proposed that a twinning arrangement be introduced taking into account:

- The number of supervisors in each district
- Geographical location within the region.

Districts which were causing some concern at LSA level would not be twinned together. (At that time one district had ten supervisors, two districts had recently amalgamated and this was twinned with two smaller districts.) Once the twinning process had been completed, the reason for audit and the process to be followed was set out.

Aim

An experienced supervisor/supervisors from a District/Trust will carry out an annual audit of supervisors within another District/Trust.

Process

1. The LSA Officer will:
   (i) produce a list of 'twinned' Districts/Trusts for audit purposes
   (ii) correspond with each co-ordinating supervisor, asking for nominated supervisors who will undertake the role of the auditors
   (iii) initiate the audit process by informing each co-ordinating supervisor of the nominated audit supervisors from the twin District/Trust, requesting them to make arrangements for the audits to be undertaken.

2. The audit supervisor will arrange to audit one or two individual supervisors each year.

3. The audit supervisor will arrange to meet some of the midwives, who are allocated to the individual supervisors referred to in 2., in order to carry out part of the audit.

4. A general discussion with the group of supervisors will follow, covering any issues raised in individual audits, which affect the group as a whole.

5. Each supervisor will have an individual audit every three years.

6. Audit reports will be submitted to the LSA on completion and at the latest by the end of December each year.

7. The LSA officer will co-ordinate the audit reports and follow up any recommendations made.

We considered that it was essential that each supervisor in the region would be the subject of an individual audit every three years in order not only to maintain a high standard but also to take supervision forward for the future.

Having now decided on the issues of 'by whom' and 'when', the next major area was 'how'.

At that time many of the maternity units in the region were using a system of audit designed by Worcester District Health Authority (1989) called SCAPA (Standards of Care and Practice Audit) and the working group requested the assistance of colleagues who had been responsible for the 'maternity' version. However, after a number of weeks it was agreed that this method was too complex and the idea was abandoned.

A simpler solution was required and having gone back to the beginning, we recognized that a simple audit could be designed, based on the 'structure' and 'process' areas of the original set of standards, i.e. did supervisors possess the documents/information etc. required to undertake their duties, and had the processes been put into place?

As we started to devise the audit tool, it soon became evident that our standards required revising and updating before further progress could be made. This work was undertaken and fortunately completed in a short period of time. Design of the audit tool then followed and when the draft was finished it was circulated for comment, minor amendments were made and the final document completed.

It was recognized that not all supervisors were experts in the field of audit and therefore training was provided by a midwife teacher (who was also a supervisor) to allow identified supervisors to become familiar with the document and for discussion to take place on the conducting of audits.

Following the training of identified supervisors, the audit procedure was implemented. It was envisaged that the audit in each district would take approximately one day to complete - giving the auditors time to complete their discussions with individually named supervisors, midwives and the remainder of the supervisors - on a group basis. Although the procedure had been agreed region wide, the working group were aware that there were, as always, a small number of sceptics.

It is accepted that if one asks any supervisor what is the biggest obstacle to her when she is undertaking her duties as a supervisor, the common answer is *time*. There is little or no recognition by managers of the time required by supervisors and therefore this important role has to be fitted in with clinical and managerial responsibilities. The group were aware that the 'time' element of the audit was going to be one of the major concerns of those auditing.

The audit procedure was implemented at the end of January 1993, but it took some time before arrangements were made by some supervisors for the audits to be undertaken.

A major difficulty had been the rapid turnover of supervisors within the region, with many of those with much experience either retiring from the NHS or leaving the region to work in other areas of the country.

During this period, the requirement for supervisors to have successfully completed the English National Board's open learning programme 'Preparation of Supervisors of Midwives' (1992) was implemented and although the principle was fully supported, it left some districts with only one or two supervisors for a long period. Under these difficult circumstances it would not have been appropriate to have visited their unit for audit purposes, or to expect them to 'audit' supervisors in their twinned district.

From receipt of the first set of audit reports, it was clearly demonstrated that the level of auditing ability varied between supervisors. This was not a total surprise to the working group. A small number of auditors had completed their task in half a day, whilst the majority had taken a full day, as expected.

The main benefits which have been recognized are:

- an improvement in networking between supervisors
- sharing of good practice.

Comments from supervisory colleagues include:

- 'Good idea - relevant information gained, but only useful in districts where supervisors are prepared to implement properly'.
- 'It assisted those [supervisors] who were not very proactive, in a non-threatening environment. Very good method - encouraged a sharing of supervision issues in comparable districts. However, there was a tendency at times for auditors to impose their views on the supervisor they were auditing'.
- 'Useful exercise - helped supervisors to look at their own standards'.

Without doubt the awareness amongst midwives of the supervisor's role, and the standard of supervision have risen significantly during recent years. How much credit we can give to the audit within the region is debatable, particularly as this was implemented at the same time as the new learning programme. However, it is still felt by many supervisors that this method of audit is more appropriate than others and for the time being we are not considering a change.

References

Ellis, R., Whittington, D. (1993). *Quality Assurance in Health Care - A Handbook.* Edward Arnold: London.

English National Board (1992). *Preparation of Supervisors of Midwives.* English National Board: London.

Royal College of General Practitioners (1983). 'The quality initiative'. *Journal of the Royal College of Practitioners,* 33, pp.523-524.

Royal College of Nursing (1990). *Dynamic Standard Setting System.* Royal College of Nursing: London.

West Midlands RHA (1991). *Standards for Supervision of Midwives.* West Midlands Regional Health Authority: Birmingham.

Worcester and District (1989). *Standards of Care and Practice Audit - (SCAPA) - Midwifery Health Authority.* Worcester: Worcester and District Health Authority.

Audit

Auditing Supervision: An Example of One Audit and General Issues Concerning Audit

Jean Duerden MBA, RGN, RSCN, RM, Cert MHS, MHSM, DMS
wrote this when Midwifery Development Project Leader at Salford Royal Hospitals NHS Trust and a supervisor of midwives. She is now LSA Responsible Officer for Yorkshire. Jean has spent most of her professional life in midwifery practice, much of it working in the community. Having completed the audit of the supervision of midwives in the North West Health Region, Jean is now involved with the ENB project to evaluate the impact of the supervision of midwives on professional practice and quality care.

Audit of supervision of midwives in the North West Regional Health Authority

The opportunity to audit the supervision of midwives in the North West Health Region was very exciting even though lying in somewhat unchartered waters. Supervision may have been around for almost a century but no one has evaluated it in any depth. In 1994 the Region was willing to spend £30,000 of Clinical Audit money on this audit. The terms of reference were clear, but the rest was up to the appointed auditor with support from a steering group to be selected by her.

Clutching the terms of reference I began my challenging year. Flushed with the excitement of a successful appointment, and the prospect of working autonomously, I set about selecting an appropriate steering group. This group of people, who included the Regional Nurse Education and Professional Development, the acting LSA Officer, a community supervisor of midwives, a midwife teacher, a clinical midwife specialist who was not a supervisor, and a midwife, proved to be a tremendous support, full of good ideas, and always willing and eager to listen.

Terms of reference

The terms of reference were:

- To undertake a systematic and independent examination of supervision of midwives in the new North West Region.
- To determine whether supervisory activities and related outcomes comply with current guidelines.

- To determine whether the arrangements for and practice of supervision of midwives is consistent and represents value for money.
- To review and, if necessary, revise the current guidelines.
- To produce a final report no later than 12 months from the commencement of the project.

A daunting task, but with all the support I had I was confident it could be done. The audit of supervision of midwives was one of many clinical audits commissioned by the North West Regional Health Authority (NWRHA). Of all those completed audits the supervision audit generated the most interest. Two conferences had to be organized to present the results of the audit to accommodate all those who were eager to hear them.

Clinical audit has occasionally had poor publicity in some areas, but the North West Health Region has taken this audit of supervision very seriously, with no suggestion that it would be taken merely as a paper exercise. Judith White, the Officer of the Local Supervising Authority (LSA), is totally committed to taking forward the recommendations of the audit.

Audit tool

For the audit tool three interview questionnaires were devised: a collective interview for all the supervisors about policies and procedures for supervision within the maternity unit; an individual interview for each supervisor of midwives; and a similar interview for midwives. The questionnaires were scrutinized by all members of the steering group. Each group member suggested amendments which were introduced into the sub-drafts. Nineteen drafts in all were written and piloted by steering group members. Excellent support and help were received from Jane Winship and Jill Steene at the United Kingdom Central Council (UKCC) and Glynnis Mayes at the English National Board (ENB) in the final stages of preparing the questionnaires. The interviews were structured to ensure that no question was open to misinterpretation and effort was made to remove the variables. In order to remain objective, the same questions were asked in the same manner.

Interviews with 385 midwives and 60 midwife teachers formed the greater part of the audit, from as few as six to as many as 18 midwives in one session. There are approximately 2950 midwives and midwife teachers in the region resulting in a sample size of 15 per cent of all midwives and midwife teachers.

The first audit took place on October 25th, 1994. There are 33 Trusts offering maternity services in the North West Region, 32 maternity units and one community midwifery service within a community Trust. Every one of these Trusts was included in the audit. As many supervisors of midwives and midwives were interviewed as could be arranged in a one day visit. Each interview took approximately 15 to 25 minutes with each supervisor of midwives, and roughly 15 minutes with each midwife, but these timings varied enormously (midwives and supervisors love having the opportunity to talk about that which is dear to their hearts). All the colleges of midwifery in the Region were also included in the audit to interview midwife teachers.

The questionnaires provided the quantitative evidence but the interviews concluded with an opportunity for comment on the supervision of midwives. All the comments were recorded and published in the final report. These comments give the audit its qualitative content and give the reader a tremendous insight into how midwives, midwife teachers and supervisor of midwives feel about supervision. The comments inevitably reflect how supervision is carried out within that particular Trust.

Audit visits

There were many interesting occurrences during the audit visits. One very unpopular supervisor of midwives sat outside the door listening (or attempting to listen) to the interviews. The midwives were aware of this and some of the confidential parts of the interview were carried out in sign language!

I was well received everywhere with generous hospitality, although on one or two occasions some hostility or suspicion from midwives was felt but it generally proved that they had a grievance to air. Many times it seemed as though I was being used as a listening post by all grades of staff. The outsider in this situation seems to be a sounding board for many anxious midwives.

The audit included interviews with 134 supervisors of midwives. There are 147 supervisors of midwives in the region, so there was involvement of approximately 91 per cent. The number of supervisors in each unit varies according to the size of the unit, but there are definite inequalities throughout the region. One large maternity unit only has two supervisors to 129 midwives. The numbers of supervisors of midwives per Trust varies from one to eleven.

Findings

Ratios

The average number of midwives per supervisor of midwives across the region is 29, which shows a great improvement since the recommendation from the UKCC of 40 maximum per supervisor of midwives was introduced (The Midwife's Code of Practice 1994, paragraph 48). Historically, the numbers have been much greater than these prohibiting effective supervision.

Individual interviews showed that two supervisors supervise only one midwife. This figure begs the question whether or not these supervisors of midwives are fulfilling their duties as supervisors. The other extreme is the supervisor who supervises 94 midwives, as well as fulfilling her management role. The level of supervision given to these midwives must also be questioned.

Grades of supervisors

In recent years, the role of the supervisor of midwives has been closely associated with management, as many supervisors have held senior midwifery positions. The audit has shown that 20 per cent of the supervisors of midwives interviewed were appointed at G grade. Sixty five per cent of the supervisors are midwifery managers and 12.6 per cent have no management role at all. The 'other' group includes: clinical specialists; a Neonatal Unit Director; midwifery advisers; Directors of Nursing and Midwifery and research and development midwives. The North West Health Region LSA recommendation is currently a minimum of grade G.

Length of service

It was very interesting to note that the average length of service is 4.4 years and only ten supervisors of midwives have served for more than ten years. The new management structures introduced by Trust boards certainly appear to have removed many long serving, senior members of the midwifery profession. Younger midwives were noted at the helm in many maternity departments, with many of the supervisors also much younger. Could this be the reason for a more enthusiastic approach to supervision? This theory was actually suggested by several of the Heads of Midwifery.

Midwife teacher supervisors

Only two of the midwife teachers interviewed are supervisors of midwives, although at the time four were registered as such at the LSA. One has since retired. The acceptability of a midwife teacher as a supervisor of midwives has been called into question recently. This was principally because they have moved into higher education establishments, out of the hospitals where they were formerly based and, of course, accessible to midwives at all times. Some of the midwives who are supervised by midwife teachers commented that they found they never saw their supervisor and felt she was inaccessible.

In another Trust, the midwife teacher who is a supervisor, is on the on-call rota with the other supervisors of midwives. She also makes regular visits to the Trust to meet with midwives and supervisors.

Areas of practice

The largest group of midwives interviewed was grade G, with the second largest group grade E. Is grade F the forgotten grade? It is noteworthy that when midwives were asked where they undertook the majority of their practice, with an option to say 'within a team', the majority consider themselves to be hospital midwives (269) with only 21 claiming to be team midwives. I know that in more than one Trust, where the interviews were carried out, all the midwives are in teams.

Only nine supervisors of midwives reported that they supervise predominantly in the community. It would now appear to be the norm for supervisors to have evenly mixed caseloads of both hospital and community midwives showing clearly that supervisors of midwives no longer supervise only midwives whom they manage.

Independent midwives

During the group interviews with the supervisors of midwives, it was identified that there were seven independent midwives practising in the Region. I was able to track down only three of them to interview, and one of those has now ceased to practice midwifery. Evidence suggests that since the RCM withdrew insurance cover for private practitioners at the end of 1994 the number of independent midwives still practising who reside in the North West Health Region has fallen to just two. There are very few problems reported with the supervision of independent midwives, which is very encouraging considering the amount of bad publicity that this topic has received in the past.

Demilew (1995) when quoting from her audit of independent midwives in 1991 states that 'All of the midwives powerfully articulated supervision being practised in a controlling, negative and obstructive way. However, two midwives spoke of their positive experience of supervision'. One must hope the two midwives were from the North West Health Region!

Practice nurses

Practice nurses who practice midwifery were found in only a third of the Trust catchment areas and there is a uniformity to the supervision offered in the majority of these Trusts. Finance could have an influence in this area. It has been suggested by at least one chief executive that fund-holding general practices should be charged for the supervision provided by supervisors of midwives from the Trust. The opinion of the midwifery officers at the UKCC on this issue is that supervision of midwives is a statutory function which cannot be avoided. Those appointed to be supervisors of midwives have an obligation to fulfil their supervision duties and charges cannot be made for this service.

Wider role of supervision

It has been interesting, and very encouraging, to learn that supervision of midwifery has an increasing role. This wider role of supervision is illustrated by the involvement of supervisors of midwives in advising purchasers of contract specifications, contributing to Trust policies, providing expert advice to outside agencies, planning schemes to empower midwives, enabling midwives to prepare for new roles and acting as a catalyst for change. As the responsibility for the LSA function transfers to the purchasers, it is likely that this wider role will expand.

Supervisory reviews

The supervisory review is one of the most important aspects of supervision and it is gratifying to learn from the audit that supervisory reviews are now commonplace and only seven supervisors of midwives interviewed do not hold them: the majority hold them annually. Cross referenced with the midwives, the majority confirmed regular reviews. More disappointing is the result from the teachers interviews where 43 per cent of midwife teachers had not had a supervisory review in the last two years, including an alarming 12 per cent who had never had a review.

Cross referencing the supervisors and midwives accounts of the duration of supervisory reviews reveals that the averages are not too far apart, nor are the minima of twelve and three minutes respectively. One can only wonder what can be achieved in three minutes, or even twelve! The quality of the supervisory review also requires assessing.

Supervisory reviews took place in a quiet place and free from interruption in all but 26 cases. Considering the fact that the majority of supervisors of midwives are busy managers, this result is very commendable and shows the importance attached by the supervisors to this time for the midwives.

There are many different expressions used to describe the reviews: annual audit, annual interview, appraisal, supervisory interview, signing of the notification of intention to practise, professional development enquiry, midwives' clinical audit, supervisors audit interview, supervisory audit interview, supervisory discussion, personal development review, supervision audit, annual meeting, midwives annual review, performance review, self review, supervisory visit, annual review of professional needs, midwives' supervisory assessment and annual professional audit (Twenty different titles in thirty three Trusts). These different titles may well reflect different views of the matter.

A sample of the forms used for supervisory reviews has been collected at each maternity department visited. They vary widely, from a simple one sided record of an interview which takes up only a few lines, to comprehensive self-review packages. The open learning pack (ENB, 1992) has made excellent recommendations for the reviews and gives examples of forms which could be developed for midwives. Many Trusts have now based their review record forms on these examples with good effect, although, it is time that some of the older ones in use are updated. Having said that, as samples of record forms have recently been requested by both myself and the LSA officer, many supervisors of midwives will no doubt be looking to carry out such an update and many so commented when handing over their forms.

Supervision of supervisors

An interesting feature of the audit was the response to the question 'Who supervises the supervisors of midwives?'. This is a very interesting perspective and surprised many of the supervisors when they were questioned. They appear to feel that they are mainly supervised by the head of midwifery or their peers, but there is little evidence of a formal structure for this in many of the Trusts. This makes one ask 'Do supervisors of midwives need supervision?'. Pettes (1979) says that 'Supervisors have needs too. They need above all to feel a satisfaction in a job well done'.

Heads of midwifery feel they have various supervisors of midwives: peers; a deputy head of midwifery; link supervisors; neighbouring heads of midwifery; a head of midwifery education; a director of nursing and midwifery. Do the link supervisors know which heads of midwifery they are supposed to be supervising? Is the LSA Officer aware of the five heads of midwifery who consider they were supervised by the LSA? Is this a formal structure? What about the two heads of midwifery who are not supervised? Do heads of midwifery need to be supervised? Faugier (1992, p.25) states

'Self-awareness is a prerequisite for selection as a supervisor... supervisors themselves should have access to either personal or group supervision in order to facilitate this process'.

Professional update

Until now, the organization of attendance at refresher courses and study days continues, in general, to be the responsibility of the supervisors of midwives, often in conjunction with the midwifery manager. There have been concerns that they would become the responsibility of the Trust training officer, and that there would be insufficient consideration of the statutory requirements of supervision. In the two Trusts where a Trust training officer does have responsibility for refresher courses and study days the statutory requirements are honoured. However, many Trusts express concern about the amount of funding available for updating.

It would appear that it is becoming common practice in many Trusts only to give the time or the money for accumulated study days. Supervisors from other Trusts complained that they were restricted in which study days could be offered to midwives because of Trust education contracts with the local colleges and universities. Where these contracts exist, only courses undertaken at those establishments are funded. Midwives who wish to attend study days on topics not available at the contracted establishment usually have to fund themselves.

As PREP is introduced, and midwives adopt those regulations, there will be no statutory reason for midwives to be treated differently from nurses and health visitors when updating. It is therefore likely that funding will be the responsibility of Trust training officers. Trust education contracts with colleges and universities will have a strong influence on any funding which may require individual contribution from professionals. Supervisors of midwives will therefore be in a difficult position when supporting midwives in their choice of update when finance will influence any decision made.

Perceptions of supervision

When considering the different perceptions of the most important functions of a supervisor of midwives, many interesting similarities were discerned. Safeguarding public interest was considered to be most important by midwives and supervisors alike, although in different quantities, and giving professional support was regarded as the second most important for every group. No one considered inspecting equipment, documentation and drug storage, to be the most important function.

This closeness of opinions is very encouraging, as is the comparison between the way in which supervisors of midwives see themselves and how they are seen by midwives and midwife teachers. The supervisors saw themselves neither as disciplinarians nor as inspectors, and few saw themselves as monitors. Only four per cent of midwives, and, surprisingly, seven per cent of midwife teachers, saw their supervisors as disciplinarians, and five per cent of each group as inspectors and monitors. Clearly the role of supporter is the most important and relevant in all the groups, which is great news for midwives and supervisors alike.

These results are a far cry from the damning article written by Beverly Beech (1993) where she refers to the supervision of midwives as victimization, and declares that disciplinary action against midwives has risen alarmingly, although there are no figures to substantiate her conclusions. She goes on to say '… many supervisors appear to see themselves as a key arm of the midwifery police force'.

One can not escape the fact, however, that, although they are few and far between, there are some supervisors of midwives who want to use supervision as a disciplinary function rather than the supporting role which it should be. One supervisor commented 'My fear is that this friend and counsellor image could be seen to reduce the effectiveness of supervision' and another 'This unit has a history of supervision being used as a disciplinary, policing role and it is difficult for the current supervisors to rectify this situation and encourage midwives to see the supportive role of supervision'. It is evident that this attitude will take a long time to overcome and eradicate.

Availability of supervisors of midwives

The availability of supervisors prompted much discussion. Many midwives said in their commentary that they find supervisors of midwives, who are also managers, to be inaccessible because of their management commitments. Despite the fact that four Trusts do not have a published on-call rota, only 24 midwives and three midwife teachers feel a supervisor of midwives is not accessible at all times.

In Trusts where there are insufficient supervisors of midwives to give 24 hour cover, arrangements are made with neighbouring Trusts and cover is shared. Some midwives and supervisors feel that this creates problems, because supervisors from other Trusts are unaware of practice and circumstances in the neighbouring Trusts. However, the majority are satisfied with the arrangement.

In a report of a ENB national workshop for supervisors of midwives (English National Board, 1983) there is a surprising entry: 'The opinion of the group was that it was not necessary for a supervisor of midwives to be on call for 24 hours a day, providing that the statutory requirements for supervision of midwives were adequately met within each Regional Health Authority. A midwife manager should always be available'.

Methods of supervision

When asked 'How do you supervise midwives's practice?' the majority of supervisors felt that in addition to the supervisory review, they also do a lot of indirect supervision by checking record keeping, visiting the wards, getting feedback from mothers and staff and auditing standards.

Observation of clinical practice is only carried out by 27 per cent of supervisors, and the time spent on direct supervision of midwives varied enormously from five minutes to sixty hours with an average of six hours according to the supervisors, four hours according to the midwife teachers and three hours according to the midwives. This shows the significance of perception again. Only a quarter of the midwives and just two of the midwife teachers interviewed had received any observation of practice within the last two years. In fact only 35 per cent of the midwives and 20 per cent of the midwife teachers had ever received observation of clinical practice since they had qualified. This observation appears to be unique to the community staff. Historically, supervisors of midwives accompanied midwives in the community on their round of home visits at regular intervals. This tradition has continued in many areas and in some, has been brought into the hospital. There was much greater emphasis on direct observation of practice in the former training for supervisors but much less in the newer preparation programme. Very few hospital staff had ever received planned observation and there is a variety of supervision in the community from supervisors accompanying midwives on their rounds, or visiting one of their clinics, to the supervisors of midwives who still visit the homes of community midwives for a supervisory visit every year. These midwives are particularly resentful of this practice.

The predominant reason for direct supervision is to supervise midwives in the community. During the interviews some supervisors appeared very embarrassed when they reported not carrying out such supervision and some gave their reason as insufficient time available rather than their finding it an inappropriate method of supervision. However, several others saw direct observation as a very false situation where the midwife performs well because she knows she is being observed. These supervisors feel that checking record keeping and supervisory reviews are much more reliable methods of supervision.

There is a noticeable difference in the approach to supervision in the community from that in the hospital. This is, of course, historical because supervision has only been relevant in the hospital situation since 1977, but nearly twenty years on we should be reaching some kind of uniformity, especially as team midwifery develops and 'Changing Childbirth' (Department of Health, 1993) is implemented.

Supervision versus management

When it comes to supervisors and midwives differentiating between the role of midwifery manager and supervisor of midwives, it may appear initially that the midwives and midwife teachers have a greater understanding of the role than have the supervisors! It must be pointed out, however, that the question was phrased differently to each group with the supervisors of midwives being asked if they had difficulty separating the roles whilst the midwives and midwife teachers were asked if they understood the difference in the roles. The latter groups probably felt obliged to say they do, rather than reveal some ignorance. In fact some midwives tried to explain the difference to the interviewer and were much relieved when told they didn't have to.

Having said all of that, as a supervisor of midwives, I can understand the dilemma faced by many supervisors. When dealing with any issue, a supervisor who is also a manager, has to think whether the issue requires a supervision or management decision or action. Module two of the open learning programme 'Preparation of Supervisors of Midwives', (Cammerloher and Sleep, 1992) seeks to assist prospective supervisors with this differentiation and is a very useful document for practising supervisors of midwives.

Joan McDowell looked at 'Statutory Midwifery Supervision - in the Hands of Midwifery Managers' in her final project report for an MSc in Research in Remedial and Caring Practice, (1993) and viewed in great depth the confusion between management and supervision. She believes that the induction course for supervisors is partly to blame for some supervisors of midwives using supervision as a disciplinary tool. Her dissertation was written before many supervisors of midwives had been prepared through the open learning programme. She believes that 'persons having the dual supervisory and managerial function can have a great advantage and could use the roles in a complementary way'. Julia Magill-Cuerden (1992) comments that the dual role can be complementary or at variance, 'The manager must deliver a cost effective service where the supervisor must ensure standards of care and quality practice'.

The issue of supervision versus management has been around for many years. The ENB workshop report mentioned earlier illustrates this. One of the eleven pages of the report is devoted to this topic when the conflict between supervision and management were discussed and 'it was felt there was no conflict when the respective roles were fully understood'.

The supervision arrangements for allocation of midwives to supervisors vary from Trust to Trust. It was particularly interesting to learn as to whether or not supervisors manage the midwives whom they supervise. In only three Trusts was this the case with all the midwives. In six Trusts this is totally avoided so that a supervisor does not supervise any midwife under her management jurisdiction (referred to as cross-supervision). In the majority of Trusts (24) there is a mixture, so just some of the midwives managed by the supervisors are also supervised by them. It is encouraging to note this trend which must encourage the differentiation between management and supervision. The introduction of team midwifery and new structures for establishing 'Changing Childbirth' has led many supervisors to reconsider their mechanisms for allocating midwives to each supervisor of midwives.

Selection of supervisors of midwives

The selection of supervisors is always very topical and there is no consensus to report here between the three groups. Midwives believe very firmly that they should have some say in the appointment of a supervisor of midwives and 55 per cent feel that election by the midwives is the most appropriate method. The 'other' category produced some interesting ideas: self nomination; nomination by midwives; psychometric testing/ development process; assessment centre; staff consultation; approval; consultation with midwives; interview with a midwife panel; criteria of skills and education; staff recommendation and finally a UKCC appointment.

The Association of Radical Midwives (ARM, 1994) produced draft proposals for the future of midwifery supervision during a working party. They believe a supervisor of midwives should be elected by her peers. She should have been practising for more than five years to be eligible and serve as a supervisor for three years. After this period she could be elected for a further three years. An allowance on top of her salary would be paid by the providing authority. No supervisor of midwives would have the authority to discipline.

The North West Region LSA have now introduced a policy whereby districts are encouraged to advertise a vacancy for a supervisor of midwives inviting self nomination by individual midwives or a consensus nomination by supervisors within the district. A detailed person specification and role specification is given to the interested midwife and she is invited to submit a curriculum vitae and piece of work in support of the application. An interview is then arranged by the appointing Trust where the midwives present their application to a panel consisting of the LSA Officer and one supervisor of midwives from the appointing Trust. The selected midwife then, of course, must undertake and complete successfully the course of preparation prior to appointment.

Just as important as selection is the deselection of supervisors of midwives, if they are unable to carry out their supervisory duties adequately. It is good to report that a procedure for this has now been established in this region.

Should midwives be able to choose their own supervisor of midwives? The supervisors of midwives are divided on this, but the majority of midwives and midwife teachers feel they should be able to choose. During the interviews even those who believe midwives should not be able to choose, feel there should be the option to change their supervisor if midwives are unhappy about their allocation.

If midwives were to be able to choose their own supervisor one could imagine various scenarios from the midwives choosing someone as their supervisor whom they felt they could manipulate, to everyone approaching just one of the supervisors and the others being left without anyone to supervise. Those who were not chosen would have to look at themselves and ask why and review their practice as a supervisor, but it would be impractical for one supervisor to supervise all the staff. The general consensus in most Trusts is that midwives are allocated to a supervisor of midwives with the option to change if they have difficulty with that allocation, although it is not easy to tell your supervisor that you would like to change.

Preparation of supervisors of midwives

The majority of the supervisors interviewed had been appointed and then prepared by an induction course, either at the Central Midwives Board or latterly at the English National Board. Nearly all of them felt inadequately prepared. Those, however, who were prepared by the new open learning course (ENB, 1992) prior to appointment, without exception felt they had been adequately prepared. This must be very reassuring to the English National Board and those who helped to write the Preparation for Supervisors of Midwives Open Learning Pack. The fact that supervisors of midwives are now mentored and prepared prior to appointment has also made a notable difference. Many supervisors previously had to deal with situations with very little understanding of the role of the supervisor and even less guidance.

Qualities of a supervisor of midwives

Glynnis Mayes (1993) wrote that the effectiveness of a supervisor of midwives depends as much on her approachability as her knowledge and decision making. It would appear that the midwives agree with her. It is without doubt the most valued quality.

Clinical experience is not far behind. Midwives feel that this is essential to give the supervisor credibility. Sympathy, wisdom and empathy were not rated highly by those interviewed.

Confidentiality was not included in the questionnaire but it was raised by many of the midwives interviewed. Many are concerned that what is told to a supervisor in confidence may be passed on, especially if it is also a manager with whom this information has been shared. This is quite disturbing. Midwives must be sure that the supervision arena is guaranteed to be confidential and information can only be shared with the midwife's consent, or if a mother and baby is at risk, and in that situation the midwife must be informed that the information has to be passed on. The supervisor may ask if she can discuss the situation with a third party to seek further advice. Supervisors are often in the position whereby they themselves do not know how next to proceed with a situation, and they need support and advice themselves.

Support for supervisors of midwives

It appears that this support is sought from a variety of sources, the most popular of which is a colleague supervisor, with the next most popular choice being the link supervisor. This vital role is well appreciated and valued by the supervisors of midwives in the North West Health Region. Now that the LSA officer is a midwife, and one with experience as a link supervisor, more supervisors feel comfortable in seeking advice from the LSA. There is, therefore, open access to both link supervision and the LSA. The Open Learning Pack is used often as a resource by supervisors of midwives, especially those who have not used it as a preparation for their role.

Who needs update?

The next issue is somewhat contentious. A practising midwife according to rule 27 of the Midwives Rules (1993) 'means a midwife who holds a post for which a midwifery qualification is essential and who notifies her intention to practise to the local supervising authority'. Neonatal unit midwives, midwife teachers and midwifery managers all fall into this category. Do they, or do they not, need to update their midwifery skills? It appears that supervisors of midwives believe that neonatal unit midwives should update, but they are less convinced about the other groups of midwives who notify their intention to practice each year.

The chosen methods of updating highlight the preference for these identified midwives to have some hands-on experience and to undertake quantified sessions working in the clinical field. The increasing use of portfolios is encouraging. The other methods of updating were: personal needs; in-service study days; their request; attend other units; study days; practice discussions, according to need; individual programmes; the role of the midwife; audit visits; informal chats; supervisory meetings; clinical placement with a mentor; theoretical input with supervision; keeping abreast with reading MIDIRS, etc.; rotation and refresher courses. One aspect which causes me concern is the fact that many supervisors feel obliged to send midwives from the neonatal units to study days and refresher courses which have midwifery practice content. This means that these midwives are not given the opportunity to up-date in their specialist area and valuable opportunities are being missed.

Midwives working in neonatal units across the region are experiencing difficulties with supervision. This problem is often exacerbated when the neonatal unit is in a different directorate from the obstetric unit. Budgetary pressures often require managers to consider carefully any updating costs. The requirements to stay on the register as a midwife involve a refresher course which can cost several hundred pounds and require a full week's absence every five years. The alternative is seven approved study days. Clinical directors have been known to say that midwives are not needed in neonatal units, only a nursing qualification is required, and are therefore unwilling to fund midwifery refreshment. Supervisors of midwives are consequently experiencing difficulties in supervising and supporting these midwives. If they offer clinical updating in the maternity unit, some managers are refusing to allow staff time out of the neonatal unit because of the demands within it.

PREP will, it is hoped, have some influence on this situation as midwives and nurses now fall into the same category as re-registration occurs for each one. It may affect updating requirements but will it change the attitude of some clinical directors to midwives working in neonatal units? I interviewed one midwife who was wearing a name badge with the title 'Staff Nurse'. When questioned she explained that the clinical director for the neonatal unit does not approve of midwives working in the unit and therefore they do not wear their correct title on their identification badges.

Support from supervisors of midwives

The majority of midwives and midwife teachers in the North West Health Region feel they get the support they need from their supervisor. There is still room for improvement and supervisors must look to their own practice to see if they are providing the necessary support, but we are on track and getting it right in most places. What alarmed me, however, is the kind of support midwives are wanting. The list grew and grew as the audit progressed and 137 different areas of required support were identified by the midwives interviewed and 54 by the midwife teachers.

The recurrent themes are change, conflict and poor practice. A few years ago, conflict with visitors and security would not have been on the list. The frequency with which concerns about the practice of other midwives was raised is also very worrying. As mentioned earlier, much has been written recently in the midwifery journals, and speakers at the ARM Super-Vision Consensus Conference referred to the 'policing' of midwives. If midwives themselves are concerned about bad practice, surely there is a need for supervision. The audit showed that the vast majority of midwives and midwife teachers agree, only three per cent of those midwives interviewed and five per cent of midwife teachers interviewed believe midwives do not need supervision.

Caroline Flint (1993) wrote that supervision 'undermines midwives' confidence in their clinical abilities' and the 'Big Sister is Watching You' article is often quoted as giving the impression that she is presenting her case against supervision. On the contrary; most of the article is very supportive of supervision. Throughout the literature search undertaken for this project there are many headlines which sensationalize the negative aspects of supervision, but when read in detail the positive aspects are invariably brought out and it is difficult to find any source which calls for the supervision of midwives to cease.

It is, however, frightening to know how much is expected of a supervisor of midwives by the midwives themselves. It is fairly obvious that all this can not be achieved as well as the other commitments that a supervisor has to meet. There is no supervisor of midwives without another role. Only one supervisor has been interviewed who receives any extra salary for carrying out her supervisory function.

The amount of support which the midwives teachers identified as needed by them is of concern. They are obviously struggling in their new academic structures to legitimize their role as practising midwives. It may be relevant to note that only 24 of the 135 supervisors of midwives interviewed supervise midwife teachers. Without exception they are Heads of Midwifery.

Clinical supervision

Another topical issue is the relationship between the supervision of midwives and clinical supervision. The majority of each group interviewed believe that statutory supervision of midwives is a good role model for other professional groups. But are not clinical supervision and the statutory supervision of midwives very different from each other?

There appears to be much confusion between statutory supervision of midwives and clinical supervision. The NHS Management Executive (1993) define clinical supervision as 'A term used to describe a formal process of professional support and learning which enables individual practitioners to develop knowledge and competence, assume responsibility for their own practice and enhance consumer protection and the safety of care in complex clinical situations. It is central to the process of learning and to the expansion of the scope of practice and should be seen as a means of encouraging self-assessment and analytical and reflective skills'. One has to admit that there is much that is relevant to the supervision of midwives in that definition.

The UKCC definition (1995) states 'Clinical supervision is a process based on a clinically-focused professional relationship between the practitioner engaged in clinical practice and a clinical supervisor. It complements, but does not take the place of formal programmes of education at pre and post registration level. This relationship involves the clinical supervisor applying clinical knowledge and experience to assist colleagues to develop their practice, knowledge and values. This relationship will, therefore, enable practitioners to establish, maintain and improve clinical standards and promote innovation in clinical practice'.

There are many comparable features, even though the Registrar's letter from which this definition is quoted is a position statement on clinical supervision for nursing and health visiting and not on midwifery. Earlier in the letter, the supervision of midwives is mentioned. 'The midwifery profession has a statutory system of supervision. Even if the law allowed for a similar development, it is not felt this would be appropriate for nursing and health visiting'.

There is a growing number of new supervisors who are undergoing a much more appropriate method of preparation, without being thrown in at the deep end to see if they sink or swim. The supervision of midwives may have a 93 year history with few changes to the requirements of the 1902 Midwives Act, but the supervision offered to midwives in the 1990s is a far cry from that of the beginning of the century and indeed from that of the 1980s. A proactive approach to supervision must continue to dominate and the reactive approach of only acting after incidents will hopefully begin to disappear.

Examples of good practice

One of the most rewarding aspects of the audit has been learning about all the good practice that is happening throughout the region and there are many excellent ideas to share. There is much more awareness of the value of good record keeping and there are many different examples of how this is monitored, from monthly random audits to supervisory meetings with midwives, where the midwives themselves evaluate the quality of record keeping.

Feedback from study days is much more encouraged. Midwives are invited to present at weekly seminars what they learned on their study days, or to present the exit modules when completing the ENB Framework. Disseminating this information is the value added to study days.

Supervisors raise their profile by having the title supervisor of midwives on their name badges and also on their door plates. They send information to GPs, purchasers, CHCs and Chief Executives to inform them about the role of the supervisor of midwives. To highlight the difference in the role, some have bleeps for the on-call supervisor of midwives distinct from the manager's bleep. Shared on-call rotas between Trusts have been established where there are insufficient supervisors of midwives to cover an on-call service for individual Trusts.

Information boards for supervision are to be found in the majority of Trusts. In-service training for midwives on supervision is now held in several Trusts, and one supervisor uses a quiz to precede this training, and another stages a roadshow.

Some supervisors of midwives have a computer data base for professional development needs, others hold critical incident seminars where incidents are discussed from a supervision perspective. One hospital uses consumer evaluation forms which are reviewed by supervisors of midwives as a yard stick for practice.

Supervision surgeries (drop in sessions in a room used exclusively for supervision which does not have a telephone) have been introduced in some Trusts, and in others there is a review of supervisory areas (audit of the midwifery practice environment).

Succession planning, regular supervision meetings with bank midwives, supervisory reviews in venues of midwives' choice, supervisory meetings for neonatal unit staff are other ways in which supervisors of midwives in the NWRHA are endeavouring to meet the current demands of supervision.

Recommendations

As a result of the audit the following recommendations were made:

1. Clarification of supervision: its function and purpose; the difference between statutory and clinical supervision; the role of the supervisor of midwives and its difference from that of manager should be encouraged and time taken for this.

2. There should be an aim within each Trust, for a ratio of no more than 25, and no fewer than ten midwives per supervisor of midwives. This should be dealt with urgently in some Trusts.

3. Those supervisors of midwives who supervise only one midwife should either increase their case load or be deselected. Supervision needs a mixed case load with realistic numbers to maintain expertise.

4. In the few Trusts where midwives experience difficulties in practising across authority boundaries, the supervisors of midwives must seek urgent discussion with colleague supervisors to resolve this problem. The 'Changing Childbirth' report (Department of Health, 1993) seeks to end fragmented midwifery care and supervisors of midwives should do everything possible to support this philosophy.

5. There should be improved liaison between supervisors of midwives across the whole region. Locality groups should be established with involvement of the link supervisors and the LSA officer when necessary.

6. The responsibility for statutory professional update, including budgetary responsibility, should stay with the lead supervisor of midwives.

7. High priority should be given to the education needs of some supervisors of midwives on preceptorship.

8. Trust Boards should seek advice from supervisors of midwives when making decisions about obstetric care.

9. The minimum grade for a supervisor should be grade G.

10. A more structured programme of supervision for midwife teachers should be drawn up and the new guidelines should address this issue.

11. The specific needs of midwives working in neonatal units should receive urgent attention and a section to address these needs included in the new guidelines.

12. The record sheets for supervision should be reviewed and revised in several Trusts using the guidelines in the open learning package 'Preparation of Supervisors of Midwives'.

13. Efforts should be renewed to raise the profile of supervision, and thus the duties of a supervisor, where appropriate.

14. Supervisors of midwives should exercise greater diligence in assessing the individual needs of midwives.

15. The areas of change, conflict, security and the impression of poor practice amongst colleagues, must be given particular attention when offering support to midwives.

16. Supervisors must examine how they themselves fulfil the role specification of the supervisor of midwives. In turn, they must inform the midwives under their supervision how their supervisory duties will be carried out.

17. Supervisors of midwives should take every opportunity to disseminate the benefits of the supervision of midwifery with other professionals. Similarly supervisors should consider the recommendations for clinical supervision to incorporate that approach into their own supervision framework and be aware of alternative models of supervision which are emerging.

18. Midwives should have the option to change their supervisor of midwives.

Conclusion

From the terms of reference given to me at the outset of the audit, it was possible to conclude that supervisory activities and related outcomes do comply with current guidelines in the majority of Trusts. Where this is not so, it would appear that the supervisors of midwives concerned are aware of the deficiencies and are anxious to address them. Arrangements for and practice of supervision are consistent and represent value for money.

There are inconsistencies, but they are few and are being addressed. It would be difficult for anyone to argue that supervision does not represent value for money, because every supervisor of midwives is appointed and paid for her clinical or managerial role. The role of supervisor of midwives is an additional responsibility. In the past, it has been suggested that the five yearly refreshment of midwives is a costly exercise; however, with the introduction of PREP the costs will be no different from those of nursing. Having identified in the audit all that a supervisor of midwives is expected to achieve, the only conclusion can be that value for money is represented.

The reliability and validity of supervision can only be questioned in those Trusts where the need for improvement has been identified. From the auditor's point of view, the high spots of the audit were interviewing midwives and supervisors who believe in the value of supervision and who receive and give an excellent standard of supervision. These midwives are obviously more confident in their practice because of the support they receive from their supervisors. It is difficult to describe but where there was obviously good supervision the atmosphere within the Trust was more positive - it was almost tangible.

The fourth term of reference was to review, and if necessary, revise the current guidelines. The LSA officer and auditor have revised the guidelines in light of the audit and each supervisors of midwives in the NWRHA has received a copy.

In conclusion I feel very positive about supervision in the region. A midwife is yet to be interviewed who is unaware of supervision and only six midwives did not know their supervisor, usually because they were newly appointed. Very few midwives believe that they do not need supervision. Fewer than expected view supervision negatively. The supervision of midwives in the North West Health Region is definitely alive and well. However, it is relevant to quote from one of the supervisors comments 'Supervision is only as good as the supervisors of midwives implementing it'.

Reflection

Reflecting on the audit it is necessary to identify mistakes made and different approaches which should be used if the audit were to be used again. I was unaware at the commencement of the audit of the problems which midwives in neonatal units were experiencing, nor those experienced by the midwife teachers. With that knowledge I would have used some means of identifying that it was a teacher or a neonatal unit midwife being interviewed and probably had a separate questionnaire for the two groups to address their problems, rather than relying on their comments at the conclusion of each interview.

The question referring to the confusion between management and supervision should have had more consistency in the midwives' questionnaire and the supervisors of midwives' questionnaire. The results from that question could be wrongly interpreted.

Audit within Trusts is a very valuable tool for evaluating the supervision of midwives offered within each Trust. Some Trusts already carry out random audits using anonymous questionnaires and the results have been acted on. The idea, from one or two Trusts, of auditing supervisory areas is also to be commended. A supervisor of midwives reviewing a work area from a supervision perspective, such as the central delivery suite where she does not work herself, can highlight many anomalies which a midwife working there all the time may not notice.

Audit has certainly, in the case of the North West Health Region, proved very valuable not just to the Region but to the statutory bodies who have hitherto had no evidence of the effectiveness of the supervision of midwives.

References

ARM Supervision Working Party (1994). 'First draft proposals for future midwifery supervision'. *Midwifery Matters*, Spring No 60, pp.26-27.

Association of Radical Midwives (1995). *Super-Vision Consensus Conference Proceedings*. Hale: Books for Midwives Press.

Beech, B. L. (1993). 'Midwife supervision or victimization?' *Modern Midwife* November/December 3:6 p.44.

Cammerloher, S., Sleep, J. (1992). *Preparation of Supervisors of Midwives: an open learning programme.* Module 2: The role of the supervisor in supporting good midwifery practice. London: ENB.

Demilew, J. (1995). 'Examples of good supervision'. in ARM (Ed). *Super-Vision Consensus Conference Proceedings.* Hale: Books for Midwives Press.

Department of Health (1993). *Changing Childbirth.* The Report of the Expert Maternity Group. London: HMSO.

Duerden, J. M. (1995). *Audit of Supervision of Midwives in the North West Regional Health Authority.* Salford Royal Hospitals NHS Trust.

English National Board (1983). *Report of a Workshop for Supervisors of Midwives on 12th - 14th October.* London: ENB.

ENB (1992). *Preparation of Supervisors of Midwives: An Open Learning Programme.* London: ENB.

Butterworth, C. A., Faugier, J. (1992). *Clinical Supervision and Mentorship in Nursing.* London: Chapman and Hall.

Flint, C. (1993). 'Big sister is watching you' *Nursing Times,* November 89:46, pp.66-67.

Magill-Cuerden, J. (1992). 'Are supervisors of midwives necessary?' *Modern Midwife* March/April 2:2, pp.4-5.

Mayes, G. (1993). 'Quality through supervision'. *British Journal of Midwifery* July/August 3:2, pp.138-141.

McDowell, J. (1993). *Statutory Midwifery Supervision - in the Hands of Midwifery Managers.* Final Project Report submitted in part fulfilment of the requirements of the examination for M.Sc. in Research in Remedial and Caring Practice.

NHS Management Executive (1993). *A Vision for the Future: The Nursing, Midwifery and Health Visiting Contribution to Health and Health Care.* London: Department of Health.

Pettes, D. E. (1979). *Staff and Student Supervision.* London: George, Allen and Unwin.

UKCC (1993). *Midwives Rules.* London: UKCC.

UKCC (1994). *The Midwife's Code of Practice.* London: UKCC.

UKCC (1995). Position Statement on Clinical Supervision for Nursing and Health Visiting Annex 1 to Registrar's letter 4.

Audit of Supervision of Midwives in the North West Regional Health Authority (1995) is published by Salford Royal Hospitals NHS Trust, DMI. Available from Salford Royal Hospitals NHS Trust, Maternity Office, Hope Hospital, Stott Lane, Salford M6 8HD at £7.50 per copy plus £1.50 p&p.

Research:
Midwives' Views of
Supervision

CHAPTER ELEVEN

Clinicians' Views of Supervision

Elizabeth M.J. Williams MSc, SRN, SCM, DN Cert, ADM
is currently Head of Midwifery for Powys Health Care NHS Trust and has been in full time midwifery practice since 1976. She graduated with a Masters degree in Midwifery from Swansea University in 1995.

Introduction

This chapter is based on the findings of a qualitative study undertaken in part fulfilment for the Degree of Master of Science in Midwifery at the University of Wales, Swansea. The work was undertaken between December 1993 and December 1994 and explores issues in supervision of midwifery from the clinician's perspective. For ease of reference, the midwife is referred to in the female gender throughout.

The concept of supervision has been enshrined in stature since 1902. It is intimately and inextricably interlinked with the history of the profession and arose from the need to protect the public from the perceived malpractice of untrained birth attendants.

During the later half of the last century, there was public concern about maternal and infant mortality whilst doctors and midwives fought for control of childbirth. An 11 year battle for legislation finally culminated in the first Midwives Act 1902, which secured for midwives the right to independent practice within clearly defined limits (Donnison, 1988). In accordance with the Act, County Councils and Municipal Corporations were designated as Local Supervising Authorities (LSAs). The LSAs were charged with responsibility for ensuring that midwives complied with the minutely detailed rules compiled by the Central Midwives Board, receiving annual notification of 'intention to practise' from midwives and investigating allegations of professional misconduct. Enforcement of these duties became the responsibility of the Medical Officer of Health, who in turn appointed Inspectors of Midwives to oversee midwifery practice (Royal College of Midwives, 1991).

This requirement for supervision has been retained and updated in successive legislation ever since. The history and statutory basis of supervision is detailed elsewhere in this book.

Background to the study

In 1990 following debate at the Royal College of Midwives Annual Conference, a commission was established to consider the strengths and weaknesses of the Nurses, Midwives and Health Visitors Act 1979 as it related to midwifery, to make recommendations to strengthen the Act and propose a strategy for achieving amendment. The working party were specifically requested to address the subject of supervision and concluded in their report, that the need for and value of it remained today. The report went on to say that 'There is no indication that it is in any way resented by midwives' (RCM, 1991: 24).

This assumption appeared to have been unsubstantiated by any research based evidence. On the contrary my own professional contact with clinical and supervisor colleagues coupled with general reading before the study provided evidence of some dissatisfaction. My experience both of being supervised and more recently as a supervisor had also led me to believe that supervision of midwifery is a valuable asset which is often poorly utilized in practice, and to the recognition that it is a powerful concept with the potential for misuse and sometimes abuse.

An extensive literature review confirmed these suspicions. The only research based evidence formed part of a, then unpublished, study of independent midwifery practice, which became available during the course of the research due to a chance meeting with its author (Demilew, 1991). The literature revealed considerable comment and anecdotal evidence and often appeared to represent polarized views, particularly about the combination of supervision and management.

Demands for reappraisal and proposals for change came largely from members of the Association of Radical Midwives (ARM), many of whom were in private practice and seemed to have suffered most from the conflicts and ambiguities involved in the concept of supervision.

Paradoxically some of supervisions' sternest critics (Beech, 1993; Flint, 1986, 1987, 1993) also acknowledged that supervision at its best can leave the midwife feeling well supported (Flint, 1993) and the public well protected (Beech and Robinson, 1992). Flint also suggested that with the introduction of general management principles into the NHS 'The supervisor of midwives may well become the saviour of our profession because her role is enshrined in statute' (Flint 1986:197).

The research described in this chapter aimed to investigate this under researched area among a group of clinicians.

Study design and methods

The research was a small scale exploratory study undertaken in a single District General Hospital (DGH). The aim was to explore clinicians' knowledge, opinions and experiences of supervision.

The specific objectives were:

1. to elicit their understanding of the statutory framework of supervision
2. to explore their views and experiences of the concept in practice
3. to establish if supervision was valued by the study subjects
4. to make recommendations relating to the findings of the study.

The aim and objectives dictated the methodology, a qualitative approach being particularly appropriate when little is known about the research question, or the research question pertains to understanding or describing a particular phenomenon (Field and Morse, 1985).

The research tool

At this exploratory stage of research, it was important to choose a research instrument that was sufficiently sensitive to explore respondents' subjective views and experiences in depth and to probe for hidden meanings.

Focused interviews thus appeared to be the most appropriate technique. In the focused interview the researcher has a list of topics he or she wishes to cover, but the interview is conducted in a conversational style (Couchman and Dawson, 1990). The research objectives formed the topic guide.

Data collection

In a qualitative study the researcher selects a small number of informants who are willing to talk and the researcher, who is in a key position, has special knowledge of the phenomenon for one reason or another (Field and Morse, 1985).

Letters outlining the study and inviting participation were distributed to all midwives by the Director of Midwifery Services. The researcher then drew a convenience sample of 12 midwives from among those on duty who were available and willing to be interviewed on the days selected for interview. The right to refuse to participate was exercised by three midwives. There was a broad range of experience among respondents from one who had very recently qualified to another who had been a practising midwife for 21 years.

The interviews

With the participants' consent, interviews were tape recorded, facilitating an ease of discussion which would have been more difficult if the interviewer were to take notes.

The interview is a special type of social relationship, which flows through the process of conversation (Denzin, 1970). However, as Denzin notes, it is not a conversation in the usual sense. The respondent may not talk, may refuse to stay within the boundaries of the interview or to avoid specific questions. A variety of techniques suggested by Spradley (1979, cited by Leininger 1985) were used to overcome such difficulties.

These included:

1.   Using broad enquiry such as 'tell me anything you would like about...'
2.   Asking general descriptive questions e.g. 'could you describe to me the qualities of your ideal supervisor?'
3.   Lead in statements were sometimes useful if the respondent had few opinions of her own e.g. 'there is a body of opinion among the profession... what are your thoughts about that?'

Data analysis

Interviews were transcribed verbatim as soon as possible after the event. The data was analysed using latent content analysis which has the advantage of retaining the richness of the data and the research context (Babbie, 1979; Fox, 1982, cited by Field and Morse, 1985). Passages and paragraphs were reviewed within the context of the entire interview in order to identify and code the major thrust or intent of the section and the significant meanings within the passage.

Multiple copies of the transcripts were cut up and sections placed in envelopes according to the developing themes. This process allows the researcher to resort the data into a different order, putting together all points about a certain topic (Riley, 1990).

The findings

Content analysis generated a total of 11 themes some of which were predetermined, others arose from the data. Sometimes respondents' own words provided the theme titles.

In order to present the findings in a logical sequence the themes were organized into three main categories. The main findings are included here.

1. Supervision in statute

This category looked first at respondents' educational experiences in relation to supervision and then went on to explore their understanding of the legislation.

a)   Educational experiences

The data provided evidence that respondents had received some instruction about supervision during their basic education programme. However, recollection of this appeared to diminish over time. They stated that little time had been allocated to the topic and the content was scanty.

Any post basic education was virtually non-existent and one informant felt that her educational experiences had provided inadequate preparation for supervision.

'I think we had half a day on it during my training and very little since...'

[Do you think your training prepared you in any way?]

'No, I don't think so at all (laughing). I mean we had a supervisor of midwives come to talk to us and she briefly outlined her role... but it was a fairly brief introduction' (6) - qualified 9 years.

However, extracts from the transcript of one interview suggested that supervision was not considered high priority by student midwives. The non verbal communication indicated that it was one of those topics one reads up before an exam and then forgets about.

No. 8: 'Yeah, we did it in our training - and I did read it up before the exams' (laughing).
Researcher: 'And you've forgotten about it since?'
No. 8: 'Obviously - because it's in the written exams... and it's a question that used to come up.'
Researcher: 'Did it make a great impression on you?'
No. 8: 'No - too busy learning about the pelvis etc.' (more laughter).
Researcher: 'Seemed more important at the time?'
No. 8: 'Well I won't need a supervisor if I don't get a job.'

The cursory attention afforded the topic both during the basic and post basic education of these midwives combined with the low priority accorded to supervision by students may be contributory factors in their poor level of understanding of the statutory framework, which was explored in the next section.

b)   'The legislation is a grey area'

Respondent's knowledge and understanding of the statutory framework proved incomplete, frequently inaccurate and on a number of occasions the legislation was described as a 'grey area'. However, most demonstrated some understanding of the origins of supervision, recognizing that it had been introduced with the first midwifery legislation and that it comprises the dual elements of protection of the public and support for the practitioner.

'The supervision of midwifery came I think - wasn't it about the 19th Century? and it's law that we have supervision... and basically it's like to supervise our practice. She's also a friend as well as a professional body.' (3)

Although midwives knew that their annual Notification of Intention to Practice is submitted to the LSA, for most of them this was a remote body. Some were uncertain about who or what this was and there was little understanding of its role and functions.

'I know that there are supervisors in the districts that they cover and that they are kind of over them... like a government body, but what the whole purpose is I'm not sure.' (8)

A number of comments indicated a limited understanding of the role of the UKCC. The question 'Who sets the standards of supervision' evoked a variety of responses, but with a little further thought some actually arrived at the correct answer.

'Umm (thinking) the actual body themselves - the RCM (thinks again) the UKCC.' (3).

Many respondents attributed their lack of knowledge about the disciplinary procedure to the fact that they had no personal experience of it.

'I don't know because I've never been through it' said No. 8.

Some understood that the supervisor has a responsibility to investigate alleged misconduct, but there was frequently an inaccurate and unquestioning belief that the supervisor has the authority to suspend from practice.

'That's the supervisor's responsibility (sounding surprised that I should ask). Who else would suspend - she's the only person who can suspend is the supervisor.' (1)

The data provided evidence of a hazy understanding of the selection, preparation and appointment of supervisors. There was some understanding of local nomination, but some respondents thought the appointment was made by the Head of Midwifery Services and others by the ENB. Some gave the correct answer, but it appeared to be more a matter of guesswork than understanding.

'I would imagine that they are proposed locally and then appointed by the supervisory board (thinks again) the local supervising authority.' (2)

A number of respondents thought that a midwife must have five years experience in order to be eligible for appointment, others thought two. Some actually indicated a total unawareness of any preparation by suggesting that there should be courses for them to go on. However, some midwives knew supervisors who had been prepared by the recently introduced Distance Learning Course (ENB, 1992) and considered this an appropriate method of preparation.

'You know supervision... is having to change and evolve all the time... X has just undergone a very intense three months... it's been validated by a University and gets so many CATS points - lots of benefits to it to be honest and in this day and age when we are producing midwives who are degree orientated - diploma orientated, then I suppose you do need a pretty solid complex course to be a supervisor.' (6)

On the whole midwives freely acknowledged their limited understanding of these important aspects of legislation and the following comments seemed a particularly apposite summary of this section.

'The average midwife I think is fairly ignorant of the Rules and what a supervisor actually does.' (6)

2. Supervision - the concept in action

Having determined respondents' understanding of the statutory basis of supervision, the researcher sought to explore their perceptions of the way it is operationalized in practice. The four themes in the second category addressed these issues. The first examined the supervisor's role in providing support for practitioners.

a) 'A safety net for us'

Some midwives in the study appeared to find the level of their responsibility to mother and child onerous and welcomed the perceived support of supervision.

> 'I think compared to nursing you are much more - you are a practitioner -you do take far more responsibility and I think it's good to have somebody there.' (8)

Supervision was a particularly valued resource in the community. The most discussed areas were home birth in unfavourable circumstances and unsupportive General Practitioners.

> 'It's somebody to go to if the GPs aren't happy with a home confinement.' (2)

> '.... a lady is demanding a home confinement and she's not very suitable ....you go to your supervisor - she supports you. It's nice to have a bit of advice.' (3)

Respondents who had worked abroad were particularly appreciative of the British system of supervision and described feeling isolated and vulnerable without it.

> 'There were still policies and guidelines.... but there was not somebody... who was there to ensure that your practice was good.' (6)

> 'I've always looked on them not only as somebody to advise, but as a safety net. If your practice is bad or unsafe in any way there is always the supervisor to fall back on and we felt very vulnerable in that situation. I'm very glad to have a supervisor. She's someone very positive in my life.' (8)

Unlike the ARM (1994) who wish to separate supervision from the disciplinary procedure, respondents in the present study saw it as an integral part of ensuring high quality standards.

> 'If you're ensuring somebody's safe practice.... the discipline aspect has got to come into it because not everybody will practise to a safe standard 100 per cent of the time.' (6)

Others made the point that if the quality of the relationship were good enough it would enable constructive criticism and facilitate personal growth and development. Some considered that effective supervision might actually pre-empt disciplinary action and protect the midwife from litigation. One actually implied that if a midwife found herself in such a position there was some failing on the part of the supervisor.

'The supervisor should have warned the midwife well before... because at the end of the day she should supervise our practice.' (3)

This seems to conflict with the notion of professional autonomy and accountability and to intimate that some midwives almost shift the onus of responsibility for standards of practice from themselves to the supervisor. Conversely one respondent made the point that clinicians are individually accountable for their own practice and questioned the appropriateness of applying disciplinary measures to force midwives to comply with the supervisor's personal philosophy of practice.

'Should somebody be really disciplined? What your supervisor is saying - you have to go along with what she says. I mean she can't make you change your practice - you're the one responsible for that.' (8)

Butterworth (1992) discussing clinical supervision in nursing suggests that in the absence of a formal model, peer support is often cited as an example of informal supervision.

Curtis (1992) contends that despite midwifery's long history of statutory supervision, an informal process of peer supervision operates as part of the cultural milieu, enabling practitioners to manoeuvre their own occupational boundaries.

This study provided clear evidence of an informal supervisory network, that appeared to have as much to do with maintaining the organizational hierarchy as with supporting colleagues.

'Being a junior midwife it's usually something I discuss with my senior colleagues... they are more likely to come and see the supervisor.' (8) - qualified 18 months.

One respondent despite 17 years experience said:

'We don't get direct supervision. It's done by the rest of the Sisters that we have.' (11)

However, despite this informal network it was felt that statutory supervision has an extra dimension that strengthens the profession.

'... I feel it gives you maybe something different. It's not another colleague who you're asking their opinion. It's a responsible person with a bit more authority to back you up.' (8)

This section demonstrated that respondents believed that supervision provides practitioners with support most notably in the community setting. There was evidence of an informal network of peer supervision, but respondents believed that statutory supervision contributes to high standards of practice and minimizes the risk of disciplinary action and litigation. They perceived the disciplinary process as an integral part of supervision with the caveat that supervision should not be used to discipline midwives who do not share the supervisors' philosophy of practice.

b)   Policies, power and supervision

Without exception respondents spoke with positive regard about their own supervisor's. However, despite this, data provided evidence of a subliminal acknowledgement of the power of supervision and its potential for positive or negative use.

Chambers 20th Century Dictionary (1983) defines supervision as 'act of supervising: inspection: control' and a supervisor as 'one who supervises; an overseer; an inspector'. Until the fourth Midwives Act 1936 supervisors of midwives were titled Inspector (CMB, 1937) and a stringent system of supervision, in reality, meant an invasion of personal privacy and value judgements about midwives' life styles. It was not uncommon for a midwife to be struck off the roll for no other reason than that she had strayed from the path of virtue (Donnison, 1988; Leap and Hunter, 1993).

An understanding of supervision as indicated by the dictionary definition and portrayed by early accounts was clearly visible in the present study.

> 'You've got to have somebody who's checking that you're doing things properly.' (1)

> 'It doesn't matter how many rules you've got [referring to Midwives Rules] some people need to have the supervisory element otherwise they would not adhere to the rules.' (4)

Although unable to offer an alternative, two respondents indicated that the title 'supervisor' reinforces this perspective.

> 'Gives the feeling that there is somebody looking over your shoulder checking on what you're doing.' (11)

There appeared to be an implicit association between supervision and a policing role and formal interviews with the supervisor were associated with discipline.

> 'One tends to associate going to see the supervisor with oh dear you're in trouble.' (6)

Respondents commented that supervision should be a mechanism for reflecting on practice, but also considered it vital for supervisors to recognize their own limitations and be open to learning.

> 'If a supervisor thinks she has nothing to learn - then she's not safe.' (4)

Batey and Lewis (1982) define autonomy in terms of structure and attitude. Structural autonomy exists when professionals are expected to exercise judgement in decision making. Midwives have structural autonomy within limits defined by statute, but may have differing levels of attitudinal autonomy.

One respondent considered that social structures within midwifery mirror those in society at large. She explained that any society functions within socially constructed boundaries and that those who fail to conform are marginalized.

'This is how we function as a society... and people who want to be very independent... very individual exists on the periphery - they are not accepted in a social group.' (4)

It may be those who display levels of attitudinal autonomy which are outside the socially accepted norm, who find themselves in conflict with their supervisors. The quality of the supervisory relationship appeared to depend on the level of interaction between individual supervisor and supervisee, which at least to an extent, depended on the midwife's own perception of supervision. Those who viewed supervision in a positive light appeared to benefit most from it.

'My supervisor has always been somebody who could point out areas where I can do extra study and develop myself... it's never been a disciplinary role... I've always thought of supervisors as someone who will take positive enquiry.' (5)

Respondents believed that policies and protocols should provide guidelines for practice rather than being too prescriptive. One referred to other hospitals in which she had worked, where they were used for policing, not only the midwives but women as well e.g. a policy that forbade breastfeeding at visiting time. She described how she disagreed with much that went on but was afraid to voice her opinions for fear of reprisals from the supervisor.

'They didn't seem to be there in an advisory or counselling role - they were just there for discipline and that was that - they weren't there for the women's benefit. [Whose benefit were they there for?] Themselves, themselves and the doctors.' (11)

She went on to say that the supervisors were very influenced by the medical staff and automatically acceded to their self ascribed superiority which she attributed in part to an unequal power distribution between the sexes.

However, despite evidence of such negative and inappropriate uses of power by some supervisors there was also a recognition of the potential to harness supervision's positive power to the advantage of both clients and the profession.

'You need to have a supervisor if you need to defend the woman against the medical staff.' (11)

'You'd have to have somebody that had actually got the power - power to make positive change.' (12)

The data in this section demonstrated the inherent power of supervision and its potential for constructive or prohibitive application. Additionally there was evidence that power is both an individual perception and a social construct. Power is often negatively associated with the combination of supervision and management. The combination of roles was discussed in the next theme.

c) Combination of roles

The topic of combination of roles was frequently raised unsolicited. Since 1974 it has been common practice to combine supervision and management. Data provided confirmation that there was confusion about the two roles and some midwives actually saw supervision as a form of management.

> 'I think there should be courses for them because... this is also a form of management.' (8)

Although respondents felt that their present supervisors were approachable, their remarks illustrated the way in which ambiguity may adversely affect the quality of the supervisory relationship.

> 'I think one of the problems with the supervisors is that they are usually your management bosses and I guess at times that could be off-putting.' (8)

However, other respondents noted benefits to the manager/supervisor combination.

> 'The managers here are also the supervisors and they are perhaps more within the unit than the managers were in nursing.' (2) - recently qualified.

Another comment appeared to concur with Lansdells' (1989) assertion that to effect change almost always requires management input.

> 'She's (the supervisor's) got to be able to influence it (the service) in one way or another. It's no good having criticisms of the unit if nothing is done about them.' (11)

There was consensus that ideally supervisors should retain clinical credibility and a view that some managers and educationalists may have lost touch with reality.

> 'I think it's possible but I don't think its ideal. (Apologises because I might be a teacher). Most teachers have very little clinical input... theoretically their knowledge is wonderful but practice is changing all the time... and I think you need a supervisor that has a finger on the pulse of changes that are occurring in practice today.' (6)

Although the clinician/supervisor combination was clearly attractive to some midwives in the study, others noted that this also has the potential for role conflicts and ambiguity of a different nature.

> 'You can't just switch off from your ward work to do the supervisor of midwife work... I think it's very difficult for somebody on the ward to be a supervisor... it must be very difficult to do both jobs.' (8)

> 'Sometimes being a manager is better... it must be quite hard to be critical and working with people at the same time.' (11)

Respondents repeatedly said that successful supervision was more to do with the individual postholder than the combination of roles.

'There are pros and cons of whichever system you use - whether you use clinical midwives or not. I feel there are advantages and disadvantages with both types. I think it depends on the individual.'

d)   The good, the bad and the indifferent

In order to gain a better understanding of the supervisory relationship the researcher sought to explore respondents' personal experiences.

Some midwives had been allocated a personal supervisor, others appeared to have chosen their own on an informal basis and yet others were about to be allocated a named supervisor.

For one respondent supervision appeared to be a total non-event. She said the supervisor was just a name to her and that she'd had very little informal contact and no formal contact with her supervisor. Although she said she would seek her out if she had problems she had never done so in three years. This was the only totally negative experience of supervision among the sample. However, 61 per cent of Demilew's informants also said that they were totally unaware of supervision before they became independent midwives (Demilew, 1991).

All respondents knew where and how to access supervision and it was generally for the midwife to initiate a meeting. Most felt that this was appropriate and that frequency of contact should be a personal arrangement between individual midwife and supervisor.

It appeared that any formal contact was initiated by the supervisor largely in response to complaints or problems. The exception to this was community midwives who had formal interviews to discuss individual professional development.

'I do when I'm out on District. I haven't whilst I've been on labour ward, but I've had formal interviews for my district supervision. [What form does that take?] Just an update.... looked at recent study days - what I'd like to do in the future - what I hope to achieve in the coming year.' (6)

Although all respondents felt able to contact the supervisor outside normal working hours, none had ever done so.

Supervision was said to be good when the supervisor offered support to midwives experiencing personal or domestic difficulties or had acted as an advocate for mothers and midwives.

Some midwives saw supervisors in a preceptorship role and one described how supervision had helped her to make the role transition from nurse to midwife.

'Although I'd been a Sister in ITU so I was used to dealing with people, the midwifery role was a new role to me and I got help and support with that when I first started here.' (1)

Another respondent described an incident where she had been concerned about a child protection issue and the supervisor had been a source of support and advice.

> 'I didn't know what to do really and the supervisor helped me - got Social Services involved - she knew the procedure.' (3)

Midwives are sometimes required to cope with situations that pose ethical and moral dilemmas and one described a situation where she finds the supervisor a source of information for the woman and counselling for herself.

> 'I find it a help in view of the increasing number of late terminations we're doing here. I feel it's right to give the women a service on the labour ward as opposed to the Gynaecological ward, but I have had occasions when I've been to the supervisor... general queries - finding out information, or generally making sure there's some follow up for the women afterwards.... and using her as a counselling service. I find that very helpful.' (11)

Midwives described supervision as 'bad' where supervision had been used to invoke organizational disciplinary procedures or when supervisors had used their powers inappropriately or ill advisedly. One, who had worked in a number of areas believed that the way supervision is operationalized in practice is greatly influenced by the culture of the organization in which the supervisor practices. She described a totally inappropriate use of supervision and abuse of the associated power.

> 'I used to get sent for regularly by the supervisor because I hadn't stuck to guidelines. I remember being sent for on one occasion because a woman was breastfeeding during visiting... and I got sent for for allowing a primip to keep her baby by her bed... I was always getting sent for but they were always things I saw as trivial... I didn't take any notice because I could never see what she was sending for me for was important - just trivia.' (11)

By exploring respondent's personal experiences this theme provided further evidence that the functions of supervision are unclear and the distinction between supervision and management often blurred. It also demonstrated that supervision can be a positive enabling experience or conversely punitive and repressive. It is because of such negative experiences of supervision that there have been calls for change. The final category discussed the future of supervision.

3. The future of supervision

Another area of interest was midwives' views of how supervision might be improved, if indeed they wished to retain it all. With one notable exception, there were few recommendations for major change. The five themes in the final category explored these.

a) 'Miss Popularity'

The ARM (1994) have proposed that supervisors should be elected by their peers for a fixed term of office. At face value this appears to be a more democratic and egalitarian approach, but whilst one or two midwives in the study were in support of the proposals, the majority were in favour of retaining the status quo. They made the point that supervision is primarily about protection of the public and should not be a popularity contest.

> 'There are times when the supervisor does have a disciplinary role and just being Miss Popularity isn't going to help in that situation, is it?' (5)

> 'If we had elected one another in the system it would be hard to be judgmental about their best friend. That's one reason why us electing supervisors wouldn't be good. Perhaps somebody should choose them for us.' (8)

There was however a strong view that there should be an effective mechanism for monitoring the supervisor's performance and deselection of supervisors who failed to achieve the required standards.

> 'Nobody's looking critically at their capabilities as a supervisor and I think there should be some way of reviewing the supervisor's role.' (11)

> 'I think if people keep being dissatisfied with the service they are offering then there ought to be a way of suggesting that supervision isn't for them.' (2)

From the data in this section it was clear that the selection of supervisors is a complex issue and any evidence for change was equivocal. It was however equally clear that midwives would welcome the auditing of standards of supervision.

b) A radical blueprint for change

One respondent had some radical proposals for change, which although representing a minority view in a small study, seemed sufficiently important to merit a separate theme.

This respondent stated that she valued the concept of supervision, but felt that it could be improved by radical restructuring.

> 'I think the whole concept of supervision is very important, but I also think the way it is structured is poor.'

She, like other respondents, had concerns about supervision and management, but also recognized that an understanding of managerial issues would be beneficial to supervisors.

Her proposals included a national core of 'Prime' supervisors appointed by the government and operating outwith the NHS. These she felt might be drawn from among the ranks of midwives who retired early. The prime supervisors would be supported by local appointees with a range of expertise who were Trust employees.

'A national core of prime supervisors throughout the country... and under her would be similar to what we've got now... would be working in the clinical field including clinical tutors... they would have to be in a position to update themselves.'

She considered that such changes might best be achieved by new and separate midwifery legislation.

It remains to be seen whether other practitioners express support for her proposals.

c) 'A professional friend'

Throughout the interviews it was evident that respondents attributed the success of supervision mainly to the individual postholder. This theme explored their concept of the perfect supervisor.

Midwives in the study had high expectations and this paragon was required to possess personal, professional and academic attributes.

At a professional level the most important qualification was broad and extensive experience in the clinical field, but current full time clinical practice was not a prerequisite.

'I would hate it to be a manager who's not working in clinical surroundings. I think it has to be people who are involved on a fairly day to day basis.' (11)

'Involved like still carrying out the midwifery care or involved with the midwifery service and the midwives working there, (doing hands on midwifery themselves?) not necessarily, but I don't think they should be too far away.' (3)

Although some respondents were quite dismissive of a need for formal academic qualifications, supervisors were expected to have an extensive knowledge in such wide ranging areas as management, education, the law and research.

'Things like counselling... the Acts - know more about the Children's Act and if you'd done the legalities in diploma studies or 997... quite current in the welfare of the state and the legislation that's coming out... as long as she had signs that she'd actually looked into research.' (3)

Personal attributes were of paramount importance. Respondents believe that the ideal supervisor should posses good communication, interpersonal and assertiveness skills. She would be mature (although not necessarily advanced in years), reflective, trustworthy, objective, kind, humble and caring, have wide vision and be open and available.

One respondent described her perfect supervisor thus:

> 'Somebody that I can go easily to and say what's worrying me - somebody you can talk to in confidence - somebody who's not too distant - somebody you can talk to and know your views will be respected.' (2)

It was clear from the evidence in this section that respondents' perfect supervisor would have a wealth of clinical experience, an extensive knowledge base, but above all the appropriate personal attributes. One respondent summed this up in the phrase 'a professional friend'.

d) Defender of the faith

Respondents speculated that in the light of the NHS reforms (NHS, 1990) and current government strategy for the maternity services (Department of Health, 1993) supervision is likely to assume increasing importance.

They commented that supervisors understand the role of the midwife in a way that is more difficult for general managers. They valued the supervisor's contribution in protecting and enhancing professional identity. In response to the question 'what difference do you see between supervision and management?' one midwife responded:

> 'The supervisor - she's got to be a midwife - somebody who does know and understand what you're talking about, whereas a manager does not necessarily have to come from the midwifery field - particularly with business management coming in - somebody on our side with the fights that we have to get ourselves recognized - with doctors and GPs, and you know our legal rights as midwives. ... She's protecting our role. It might get eroded like so many American systems.' (8)

Another respondent provided first hand evidence to support such an argument. She referred to the time she was abroad and described an incident where her non-midwife manager had considered it appropriate for a health visitor to deputise for a midwife and went on to explain that, without supervision, she feared the same situation could arise here.

> 'Especially with going Trust. It would be very easy for people to see it (midwifery) as nursing... in these days of business management and cost cutting - the supervisor can bring a stronger argument and in a different capacity than the ground floor worker... because if your manager says do something you're in a difficult position and we were in a very difficult position for a while.' (5)

With the introduction of an internal market in health care and with the emphasis on client choice midwives both independently and as NHS employees have the opportunity to compete for purchaser contracts. The midwives in this study believed that the supervisors' role in maintaining a high quality service makes her a key player in securing, for midwives, a satisfying share of the market.

'It could become a much more important role... if midwives are going to be the lead practitioner the supervisor must ensure that the midwives in her area are practising as the public want - at the end of the day if they don't want us we're lost... she could have a more important role.' (11)

The midwives interviewed in this study believed that the supervisor has a central role in maintaining the unique and separate identity of the midwifery profession and in ensuring a high quality marketable service.

e)   In praise of supervision

There was no evidence in the data that respondents wished to abolish supervision. On the contrary there was considerable strength of feeling in favour of retaining it.

'I certainly don't think we should do away with supervision.' (4)

'I wouldn't want to be without supervision. It's there as a safety net for us... and without supervision I'd find it very hard.' (7)

One respondent asserted that because of the midwife's role as an autonomous and independent practitioner, supervision is still relevant in protecting the public.

'I think supervision is vital... at the end of the day there has to be some method of protecting the patient - I think supervisors are essential... I would fight for that. I agree that we are autonomous and that we are regaining our independence - that we are practitioners in our own right, but I think that in itself leads to greater danger in some respects and I do think we need a framework of supervision.' (6)

The data in this final theme demonstrated that midwives in the study hold supervision in the highest regard and would actively seek to retain it.

Discussion

The study suggested that among this group of midwives, education in relation to supervision was poor. Respondents perception was that time allocated to the topic during basic education was minimal and the subject barely addressed at all during post basic education programmes. There may be a number of explanations for this unsatisfactory situation. Supervision was taught either by supervisors whose teaching skills may have been inadequate or by educationalists whose own supervisory experiences may have been poor.

However, there is a danger in making the assumption that teaching and learning are synonymous. There was evidence that supervision was not a priority for student midwives. It only became important if and when the student qualified and commenced midwifery practice.

Midwives interviewed in the study had a limited knowledge and understanding of the statutory framework for supervision. This poses two problems. Some midwives appear to be arguing for a change in legislation (ARM, 1994), but this is an issue that affects all midwives, and a thorough grasp of the issues is required to make an informed contribution to the debate.

Secondly, successful supervision is based on a partnership between supervisor and supervisee and a basic understanding of the statutory framework is required to enable the supervisee to make an effective contribution.

That midwives can have such widely differing experiences of supervision is worrying. At its best, supervision leaves midwives feeling secure and supported and the public protected from poor standards of practice. At its worst, it constrains practice, inhibits woman focused care and brings both the concept and the profession into disrepute. Midwives in the study believed that there should be some method of monitoring standards of supervision and deselecting supervisors who fall below the required standard. The study also highlighted the desirable qualities we should be seeking when considering the selection of supervisors, but on the whole respondents did not wish to see supervisors elected by their peers.

The data provided evidence of an informal network of peer supervision and it is tempting to assume that because it exists, midwives must value it and this may be so. However, the fact that it appeared to operate on a hierarchical basis leads to the suggestion that it has an alternative significance.

Midwifery is influenced by the culture of the organization in which it is practised and Curtis (1992) has suggested that such informal supervisory networks are employed by midwives in an effort to shake off the bureaucratic and medical constraints constructed by such organizations. All professionals will at some time wish to seek advice, but by seeking it from the 'next up' in the chain of command midwives may be reinforcing the bureaucratic constraints they seek to shake off. Hugman (1991) has argued that power is socially constructed, but because it is also socially located it may have the appearance of consensus. Such hierarchical structures may have been absorbed into the cultural norms, to the extent that midwives are totally unaware of their effect.

Confusion about the functions of supervision and management has led to the use of, or perceived use of, supervision (a professional activity) to reinforce bureaucratic control and leads some to recommend separating the roles (Isherwood, 1988; Royle, 1994; ARM, 1994). This study confirmed the confusion that exists and suggested that some midwives saw supervision primarily as a form of management. Clearly individual perceptions and misconceptions of the role will influence a midwife's relationship with her supervisor. If the supervisor is seen as a 'wise sage' she will be approached as such. If on the other hand she is seen as an agent of bureaucratic control, the clinician is unlikely to look to her for support and guidance. However, some respondents noted benefits of combining the roles of supervision and management. The ability and authority to effect change in practice and the organization of care was more easily achieved when the manager was also a midwife and the supervisor of midwives. Midwives also recognized that other possible combinations whilst being advantageous in some respects, would also have role conflicts and ambiguities of a different nature.

There was sound evidence that respondents considered supervision to be important, not just to the individual, but for the midwifery profession as a whole. They believed that it gives the profession a strength and security that will become increasingly important in the light of the NHS Reforms and in supporting and driving recommendations for change in maternity services. With one notable exception there were no recommendations for major change.

Implications for the profession

This was a small scale exploratory study and therefore context specific, so no claims can be made for generalization. However, the study contributes to our understanding of the concept and a number of implications arising from the findings are suggested here.

The aims of supervision are laudable, but it appears that they are sometimes attenuated by the way it is implemented in practice. The power of supervision should not be about limiting practice, but about enabling it, not about constraining practitioners but about empowering them. Evidence from this study that this can and does happen suggests that the legislation is not inherently flawed. It seemed to suggest that it is possible to work within existing legislation, supporting good practice to improve standards, whilst maintaining final sanctions to deal with professional misconduct.

There remains a perception of supervision in its historical sense of authority and control which appears to be reinforced by the title. Perhaps this merits attention if the profession wishes to ensure that supervision is a positive enabling experience. This and the obvious uncertainty about what exactly supervision is suggests a need to clarify the concept and define its component parts.

The study indicated that selection of supervisors is not a simple matter and changes should not be introduced lightly. There are strengths and limitations both to appointment and election. Clearly no system would be foolproof but an acceptable compromise might be to invite nominations from a variety of sources. Candidates could then be screened by a panel of assessors, paying attention to the desirable personal, professional and academic attributes.

Perhaps the time has come to stop arguing about the combination of roles and to acknowledge that each possible combination has its own particular strengths and weaknesses. Nominating supervisors from a range of backgrounds would bring a wealth of knowledge and experience to the role and help to mitigate the negative aspects of each combination.

If the profession chooses to invest the power of supervision in an individual, there is an obligation to ensure that it is appropriately and wisely used. There appears to be an urgent need to define acceptable standards of supervision and ensure some consistency of approach. A first step might be to identify, disseminate and promulgate examples of good practice and then to instigate a mechanism for auditing these standards and dealing with supervisors who fail to attain them.

Kirkham (1994) has suggested that clinicians might choose their supervisors from a number of appointees and this would offer one solution to the problem of conflicting philosophies of practice. Another might be for the profession to identify and adopt a unified philosophy of practice. Whether or not this is realistic or desirable is open to debate.

An informal supervisory network, operating on a hierarchical basis, may reinforce socially constructed constraints on midwifery practice. Scott (1966, cited by Davis, 1992) contends that a professional carries out a complete task and is loyal to a company of equals, seeking no higher position within the organization. If midwifery aspires to be a profession, career structures should be flattened, midwives carry their own caseloads and work in small teams or group practices. When we have dealt with our own socially constructed constraints, it may be easier to deal with these imposed by other professions. If we want supervisors who are strong and professionally courageous, we must be grooming them in the ranks of the profession. Without this grounding, the cycle of poor supervision will be perpetuated.

Midwives' education in relation to supervision appears to be a critical factor. It should be introduced during basic education and become an integral part of the midwife's life long education and learning. The focus should be directed not just to giving information, but to exploring the way supervision impinges on practice.

The study concluded that supervision in midwifery is held in the highest regard by midwives and is a concept that should be retained and updated.

References

Association of Radical Midwives (1994). 'First draft proposals for future midwifery supervision'. *Midwifery Matters*, No.60, Spring pp.26-27.

Babbie, E. (1979). *The Practice of Social Research*. 3rd Edition California: Wadsworth Publishing Co. cited by Field, P., Morse, J. (1985) *Nursing Research - the Application of Qualitative Approaches*. New York: Chapman and Hall.

Batey, M., Lewis, F. (1982) 'Clarifying autonomy and accountability in nursing service'. *Journal of Nursing Administration* Sept. pp.13-18.

Beech, B. (1993) 'Midwife supervision or victimisation?' *Modern Midwife* Vol.3, No.6, p.44.

Beech, B., Robinson, J. (1992) 'Hard labour' *Health Services Journal* Vol.102, No.5286, pp.26-27.

Butterworth, T. (1992). 'Clinical supervision as an emerging idea in nursing', in Butterworth, T., Faugier, J. (Eds). *Clinical Supervision and Mentorship in Nursing* London: Chapman & Hall.

Central Midwives Board (1937). *The Midwives' Acts 1902 - 1936*. London: Spattiswoode & Ballanstyne & Co. Ltd.

Chambers (1983). *Chambers 20th Century Dictionary*. Edinburgh: Chambers.

Couchman, W., Dawson, J. (1990). *Nursing & Health Care Research - A Practical Guide*. London: Scutari Press.

Curtis, P. (1992) 'Supervision in midwifery practice' in Butterworth, T., Faugier, J. (Eds) *Clinical Supervision and Mentorship in Nursing*. London: Chapman & Hall.

Demilew, J. (1991) 'The struggle to practise - a sociological analysis of the crisis within the British Midwifery Profession'. *MSc Dissertation* South Bank Polytechnic

Denzin, N. (1970). *The Research Act in Sociology*. London: Butterworth.

Department of Health (1993). *Changing Childbirth*. London: HMSO.

Donnison, J. (1988) *Midwives and Medical Men*. London: Historical Publications Ltd.

English National Board (1992). *Preparation of Supervisors - Open Learning Programme*. London: ENB.

Field, P., Morse, J. (1985). *Nursing Research - the Application of Qualitative Approaches*. London: Chapman & Hall.

Flint, C. (1986). *Sensitive Midwifery*. Oxford: Butterworth Heinneman.

Flint, C. (1987). 'Conflicting allegiances' *Nursing Times* Vol.83, No.5, p.24.

Flint, C. (1993). *Midwifery Teams and Caseloads*. Oxford: Butterworth Heinneman.

Fox, D.J. (1982). *Fundamentals of Research in Nursing* (4th edition) Connecticut: Appleton Century Crofts cited by Field, P., Morse, J. (1985). *Nursing Research - the Application of Qualitative Approaches*. London: Chapman & Hall.

HMSO (1990). *NHS and Community Care Act*. London: HMSO.

HMSO (1979). *Nurses, Midwives and Health Visitors Act*. London: HMSO.

Hugman, R. (1991). *Power in Caring Professions*. London: Macmillan.

Isherwood, K. (1988). 'Friend or watchdog?' *Nursing Times* Vol.84, No.24, p.65.

Kirkham, M. (1994). 'Supervision - a contribution to the debate' *Midwifery Matters* No.60, Spring 1994, p.27.

Lansdell, M. (1989). 'Friend and counsellor' *Nursing Times* Vol.85, No.28, p.76.

Leap, N., Hunter, B. (1993). *The Midwife's Tale*. London: Scarlet Press.

Riley J. (1990). *Getting the Most from Your Data - A Handbook of Practical Ideas on How to Analyse Qualitative Data*. Bristol: Technical & Educational Services Ltd.

Royal College of Midwives (1991). *Report of the Royal College of Midwives Commission on Legislation Relating to Midwives* London: RCM.

Royle, N. (1994). 'Supervision - Where do we go from here?' *Midwives Chronicle and Nursing Notes*. Vol.107, No.1275, pp.137-138

Scott, W.R. (1966). 'Professionals in bureaucracies: areas of conflict.' in Volmer, H., Mills, D. (Eds) *Professionalism Prentice Hall*. Inglewood Cliffs cited by Davies, C. (1992) 'Professionals in bureaucracies: the conflict revisited.' in Dingwall, L. R., Lewis, P. (Eds) *The Sociology of Professions*. London: Macmillan.

Spradley, J. (1979). *The Ethnographic Interview*. New York: Rinehart & Winston pp.78-79, 85-87, 155-172 cited by Leininger, M. (1985). 'Ethnoscience and companential analysis' in Leininger, M. (Ed). *Qualitative Research Methods in Nursing*. London: Grune Stratton.

CHAPTER TWELVE

Midwives Perceptions of the Role of a Supervisor of Midwives

Cathy Shennan BN, SRN, HV, DN, SCM, ADM, MSc, PGCEA
is currently working as a Senior Lecturer at Anglia Polytechnic University. She trained as a midwife at Newcastle-upon-Tyne and has worked as a lecturer at Kings College Hospital. She has also successfully completed her Masters Degree in Midwifery with the University of Manchester.

Introduction

The role of supervisor of midwives is unique to midwifery and is enshrined in statute. At the very heart of supervision is the safety of mother and baby. The Ministry of Health (1937) pointed out that:

> 'an inspector of midwives should be regarded as the counsellor and friend of the midwives, rather than a relentless critic, and should be one who is ready to instruct the midwives in the various points of difficulty which arise from time to time in connection with their work and make them feel that there is always someone to whom they can look for sympathetic understanding of the laborious nature of their profession'.

Whilst the term 'inspector' has changed to 'supervisor' what was stated then is still equally applicable today. This theme is echoed in the May 1994 edition of the 'Midwives Code of Practice' (UKCC, 1994):

> 'Your supervisor of midwives should give you support as a colleague, counsellor and advisor. This should be developed in order to promote a positive working relationship which is conducive to maintaining and improving standards of practice and care'.

It is perhaps also worthwhile looking at the definition of clinical supervision as given by the NHS Management Executive (1993):

> 'A term used to describe a formal process of professional support and learning which enables individual practitioners to develop knowledge and competence, assume responsibility for their own practice and enhance consumer protection

and the safety of care in complex clinical situations. It is central to the process of learning and to the expansion of the scope of practice and should be seen as a means of encouraging self-assessment and analytical and reflective skills'.

Supervisors of midwives, however, also have a responsibility to inform and advise the Local Supervising Authority (LSA) where there has been a case of alleged misconduct. Suspension from practice can only be authorized by the LSA when it has reported the midwife to the Statutory Body for investigation, or when a referral has been made to the Professional Conduct Committee or to the Health Committee of the UKCC. Where the supervisor of midwives is also a manager however, she can suspend a midwife from duty, as an employee, in cases of alleged misconduct in accordance with the employer's local disciplinary procedures. It may be considered that these latter responsibilities of a supervisor are likely to militate against a midwife discussing with a supervisor any weaknesses or problems she may be experiencing with her work. This is particularly so in the current climate of recession with the ever present threat of redundancies.

The aim of this research is to learn about the nature of supervision from a practising midwives' perspective; to explore the experiences that midwives have had with supervisors; to discover the 'insider view'; to learn to see the world from the eyes of the person being interviewed; to walk in their shoes and to examine and analyse their perceptions. I wanted to learn what supervision meant to the midwives and to explore as Lincoln and Guba (1985 p.258) state 'the norms, attitudes, constructions, processes and culture that characterise the local setting' in relation to supervision. I wanted to learn how the written guidelines had been translated into practice. It is hoped the results of this study may inform future curriculum planning for 'Preparation of supervisor of midwives' courses.

No published research has been located on this subject. There is no reference to supervision in midwifery in the 1994 edition of the Midwifery Research Database (Simms et al, 1994), nor is there any reference to supervision of midwifery in the classic text 'Effective Care in Pregnancy and Childbirth' (Chalmers, Enkin and Keirse, 1989) or the Cochrane Collaboration Database (Enkin, Keirse, Renfrew and Neilson, 1995), although supervision of midwifery does not lend itself well to quantitative randomized controlled trials which the latter tends to focus on. This is, therefore, a unique and necessary piece of research. All my data were collected before looking at the literature so as not to bias my findings.

As an experienced midwife and lecturer in midwifery, my own experiences of supervisors of midwives had been negative up to the point when I commenced this research. I had only once had a supervisory interview. I felt the supervisor was not up to date with current research and criticized practice which was based on current research because it conflicted with midwifery policies dictated by consultant obstetricians.

Study design

This was a qualitative survey within the naturalistic paradigm, which focuses upon an 'emic' or insider perspective. The design of the research was emergent, not preordinate, it was moulded by the multiple realities that the volunteer midwives shared with me and the context within which they worked.

The sample

Midwives were invited to participate if they felt 'they could make a useful contribution to the research'. As such there could be no a priori specification of the sample - it simply could not be drawn up in advance. As the qualitative research process was extremely time consuming, both for the collection and analysis of the data, and because of the limited period of time involved for the conduct of this research it was intended to keep the number of the sample small - a maximum of twelve midwives were recruited. Midwives were only included if they had a minimum period of one year's experience after registration. I obtained all the names of the midwives in the area from the senior supervisor's secretary. I decided to exclude those midwives who were on maternity leave, who were on long term sick leave and bank staff. In total 116 midwives were written to. I wrote out a personal letter to each midwife and included an informed consent form which was based on the material in Field and Morse's book (1985, p.45). Fifteen positive responses were received. Other responses were received from midwives thanking me for inviting them to participate but declining as they felt they had nothing useful to contribute.

Data collection

I asked the midwives when and where they wanted to be interviewed. I tried to conduct interviews in off duty time. Focused interviews were tape recorded which provided high fidelity data. Tape recorded interviews further facilitated seeking the words of the midwives that I was studying, so I could understand their situation with increasing clarity. Tapes were destroyed before the data were published. The questions I tended to ask were mainly of the 'grand tour' type (Spradley, 1979). For example, 'I'm really interested in your experiences of supervisors of midwives, would you like to share some of them with me?'. The object of this 'orientation and overview phase' according to Lincoln and Guba (1985) was to get a grasp of what the midwives considered important so that it could then be followed up and explored in more detail. The midwives spoke very spontaneously and seemed to enjoy talking to me. Some of the midwives talked non-stop for one and a half hours. As I became more adept at interviewing I was talking less and less and the midwife was talking more and more. The following probes worked very well:

- 'I was interested in what you were saying about... can you tell me more about that?'
- 'Can you give me an example of what you are talking about?'
- 'What do you mean by...?'

Two pilot interviews were conducted. This enabled me to correct problems such as not being able to hear what was said on the tape by placing the tape much closer to the midwife in the main study. It also helped me to develop the ability to ask probing questions, to follow the lead of the midwife and at the same time try to avoid becoming side tracked.

Data analysis

Continuous data analysis occurred, so that every new interview was informed by what had gone on previously. Content analysis was used to analyse data; a process aimed at uncovering embedded information and making it explicit. This involved a process of 'unitizing' and then 'categorizing'. Unitizing is a process of transforming raw data into units which allow precise description of relevant content characteristics. The unitized data is then drawn into categories that describe the context from which the units were derived.

Credibility

Member checking was used to establish credibility. Full transcripts of interviews with five of the midwives were posted to them. They were asked to confirm whether or not they felt this was an accurate record of the interview and invited to make additional comments. All five midwives responded in writing confirming that the interviews were an accurate record. An audit trail was also kept to establish credibility. This included a research diary including reflections on learning and discussions with my research supervisor, written correspondence to the chairman of the local research ethics committee and written permission from the senior supervisor and chairman of the ethics committee to undertake the research.

Ethical issues

Two supervisors in this inner city area had been approached on an informal basis in order to obtain their verbal agreement to proceed. A copy of the research proposal was then sent to the chairman of the local research ethics committee and to the senior supervisor of midwives in the area under study. It was stated that midwives would remain anonymous. The chairman of the ethics committee stipulated that trained midwives should opt in and that written permission from the senior supervisor would need to be obtained.

Since the design of this study was emergent it was not possible to foresee problems occurring. Though given the option, none of the midwives withdrew from the research. Special care has been taken to prevent raw and processed data being linked with a specific informant. Names of midwives were not included on transcripts. Identities of midwives throughout this chapter are disguised.

Characteristics of the area

Although I had invited the participation of both midwives in independent practice and in the National Health Service, all those who volunteered worked for the National Health Service. Some of them worked in a consultant obstetric unit, others in GP units, and yet others, probably the majority, worked in the community. These midwives were not recently qualified and they had years of experience. Most of them had worked in the same area for many years. Group practices in midwifery or team schemes had not yet been introduced in this area. Two of the midwives had experience of acting as supervisors of midwives. This study seemed to attract many of the midwives in the area with advanced professional education.

Findings

The main category which developed from the data was one of support. All twelve midwives spontaneously spoke about this subject. The examples cited identified a continuum between being very well supported on the one hand to being very poorly supported on the other. There were various dimensions to being well supported (see Table 12.1) and being poorly supported (see Table 12.2).

Good support meant:

- That the supervisor had the strength of personality and knowledge to solve problems
- That the supervisor took concerns seriously.

Table 12.1: Good support

Poor support meant:

- That a midwife had no one to turn to in times of crisis
- That midwives were suspended over the telephone and there was no face to face contact
- That the supervisor lost perspective of what was important
- That supervisors pointed fingers and apportioned blame
- That supervisors did not establish the facts prior to suspension
- That midwives were told off for something they had no control over
- That midwives were not given the opportunity of explanation
- That midwives did not know the reason for suspension
- That supervisors were oppressive and used their power destructively
- That midwives were treated as children
- That midwives were not allowed to make their own decisions
- That supervisors down-loaded their problems onto midwives
- That midwives were unable to talk through their feelings
- That supervisors undermined a midwife's confidence to practice
- That supervisors prohibited access to medical records
- That midwives were expected to stick to rigid protocols
- As a result midwives went underground.

Table 12.2: Poor support

Support

When midwives spoke of good support they spoke of a supervisor being able to take on situations that they were unable to cope with themselves, that they themselves found stressful. Fiona, a community midwife described a current problem and how a previous supervisor would deal with problems. The use of metaphor by midwives throughout this section is significant:

> 'Some of the antenatal care they (the mothers) were getting was from the practice nurses who were not midwives. So dealing with these GPs on your own is extremely difficult because they, the Senior GP, uses a verbal aggression in a way that I have never known a so called professional to use. He treats midwives as silly women who really all they need is a good man basically and that would solve all their problems.... When we had Miss Baron, Miss Baron was a midwives supporter at all times and we knew that in a situation where midwives were being sidelined and the women were not getting the midwifery input they should have done, she would come in like a bat out of hell and she would do it through force of personality as much as through anything else, and her knowledge was phenomenal - she would almost frighten people into changing their behaviour but we don't have a Miss Baron'.

Support for Fiona meant that the supervisor had the knowledge and strength of personality to solve problems when midwives were not getting the recognition they deserved. The use of metaphor is powerful, it suggests that the supervisor responds very quickly, not with assertion but with aggression.

Support from the supervisor also meant that concerns were taken seriously. An example of this is given by Carol, a community midwife:

> 'It was over a particular time of stress. These things are always dangerous. You have sickness, holidays, a busy period coinciding, that is when it always happens. In Tarant it arose a couple of times, where we had been trying to cover shortages of staff in the hospital, as well as being stressed and busy on community, and feeling also that our competence for working all day as well as working all night, was putting ourselves at risk of making mistakes. And when we first had a meeting about that was a long time ago when Miss Baron was here, and she was actually very supportive and took our concerns seriously and came to a meeting and talked to us - and the situation seemed to resolve itself.'

Support for Carol meant that the supervisor showed genuine interest and concern by calling a meeting during troubled times. Support meant that she took the time and trouble to talk to the midwives and took their concerns seriously and acknowledged that there was a problem. She showed an appreciation for their feelings and had the ability not only to listen but take on board what the midwives were saying.

Poor support

Suspensions

Midwives talked about supervisors not establishing the facts prior to suspension and suspensions being made over the telephone. (It is perhaps worth noting again that where a supervisor of midwives is also a manager she can suspend a midwife from duty in accordance with the local disciplinary procedure.) Midwives spoke about situations when midwives had no one to turn to in times of crisis; all support networks having been deliberately severed. The following incident described by Teresa illustrates these points. She recalled an incident where a midwife had accidentally given a single dose of an oral antibiotic to the wrong mother on a postnatal ward, had not recorded the administration of the drug, nor reported the error.

> 'A couple of days later this lady said to the discharging midwife "oh I had that antibiotic one day, that will be all right won't it?" The discharging midwife was in a terrible dilemma - what should she do?. She decided, I think quite rightly, to pass it on... mitigating circumstances (for the midwife who made the error) were that she had also been dealing with a lady with a stillbirth and had been up and down all day and had become very distressed about it but had not let anyone know. She said she should not have been made, and in a way I agree, to look after the others when there was a lady that had a stillbirth that needed a lot of care, which is right. But what really upset me was that she was suspended over the phone - told not to come onto the property and was off for - the suspension was not lifted for three weeks and then she was off for stress - which often happens. I just thought that was a bit hefty for what she did. I was told when I questioned it - you know I felt it was a learning exercise for me to question it anyway - I was told because she covered up the incident they did not want her in contact with any of her colleagues. This was on the phone. She was on the phone to me. That was another thing I find very difficult. She was a) a neighbour almost and b) she was ringing me up and I had to say to her look I can't do anything for you, you must contact the steward in the college. But thought it was a bit hefty for what she did and in the end when they had it all the mitigating circumstances got her off if you like. You see managers don't have to answer for using the wrong - not that a manager ever admitted to be being heavy handed but they don't have to answer do they? - for doing something heavy handed.'

There was no one familiar to whom the troubled midwife could turn to for help. There had not been full exploration of mitigating circumstances before the decision to suspend was made. The decision to suspend was made known to the midwife over the telephone and not in a 'face to face' interview. There is also the suggestion here that suspension is not an isolated occurrence, it is in fact quite usual for midwives to go off sick with stress, 'it often happens', once the suspension is lifted.

Similar themes were identified by Tanya who was just completing her Diploma in Professional Studies Midwifery. Tanya described how she had been 'suspended from practice' by a supervisor. She had admitted a woman expecting her second baby to a GP unit. The woman was having irregular contractions and the midwife did not feel labour was established. The membranes were still intact and the cervical os was between three and four centimetres dilated. The mother had previously had a retained placenta and this is why she had been booked at a consultant obstetric unit some twenty minutes drive away. Tanya suggested to the mother that her husband should drive her to the consultant obstetric unit. The mother delivered en route to the consultant obstetric unit in the car. The story was published in the press. Someone had to take the blame. The next day Tanya was suspended over the telephone by the senior midwife:

> Researcher: 'And how did you feel about that?'
> Tanya: 'Well I was shocked, I was thirty four weeks pregnant and two days later I was going on maternity leave and I was just shocked, absolutely shocked, I just couldn't believe it, it was like someone had hit me.'

Tanya was never told the reason for the suspension either verbally or in writing. She was not told what alternative action she should have taken in the circumstances. She did not even know who made the decision to suspend her. The responsibility for suspension appeared to be diffused amongst a number of different people. She said that instead of having to rely on what she had heard through the grape vine, it would have been better if she had been told.

> 'I think the problem is that because when you work you like to trust people, you like truth, something that happened to me that I just could - because I had not expected to have suspension from. As far as I was concerned I had made a decision, had stuck by that decision, like you make thousands of decisions every day, thousands of decisions and all of a sudden by no fault of my own something had happened and I was being blamed for it - which seemed very unfair, I think particularly so, in the sense that I felt aggrieved in the fact that I was pregnant and two days later I would have gone on to maternity leave. Nobody had actually come to me in the unit to offer any support, it was more or less you are in the wrong. It had not been investigated thoroughly and yet I was sent home and not allowed back onto Trust premises. It was a big shock to the system but when you are pregnant it is even more. It just makes you feel that why do you bother at times, why do you bother trying your best, giving your best care and then treated not very fairly?'

Tanya went on to describe how it affected her practice,

> 'the problem is then that it knocks your practice because you are encouraged to make decisions upon what experience you have and what knowledge you have... the problem is then with an incident like that you lose trust... yes, it would be natural to lose trust in supervisors, yes.'

Tanya did not feel supported by her supervisor,

> 'The problem was supervisors are then management and these are the people who are saying that I was wrong and who were investigating so I was out on a limb in a sense.'

She was in fact supported by the woman's General Practitioner.

'The next day I phoned (the GP) and he could not talk for a few seconds - he was so shocked at what had happened... and he said was there anything that he could do to help support me - anything at all - and he suggested "will I write?"'

Tanya described the nightmare she had been through. The worry, suffering and stress, she described how she was unable to sleep at night and how she cried most days.

'I was left questioning everything really - how far were they going to take it? Are we talking about me losing my job? You imagine the worst scenario really... it seemed, it was just very dramatic... I had heard they were going to try and the objective was to get me for gross negligence or gross misconduct, I was quite amazed really, it was just really stupid you try and relate it to me being suspended and talking about this line of action. It did not compare with the incident it was just like it was way over the top.'

Tanya was suspended for two weeks and had a hearing at the end of it. She was accompanied by an Industrial Relations Officer from the Royal College of Midwives. She was pleased he came because she felt he provided a lot of support.

'Fortunately the Directorate Manager Tessa had actually attended as well, she had one of the letters from the GPs... I was asked a few questions during the hearing. I left the room whilst they discussed the incident and I went back in and they said they were really quite happy and I could not have known she would have delivered so soon and it was just one of those things.'

It left Tanya feeling very angry and bitter.

'I believe that because I am accountable as a practitioner, midwives are also accountable as supervisors. The decisions that they make - I feel - that I was suspended and the outcome of it was they say I was not to blame, it must reflect on who made that decision - they are accountable for making that decision. They are also accountable for the decision that they put me in at that stage, suffering really. What reflection is it on them who made that decision? They were heavy handed with me but I don't know what the outcome was with them. You think well OK perhaps they have learned from experience perhaps not - but then does it take a lot of suffering from somebody for them to learn from experience...? You have to come and talk to someone face to face in an important situation such as suspension. You have to come and talk to someone face to face because if you are going to suspend someone as I have said previously, you have to explain why you are suspending them... if you are going to make such a big decision as that you have got to have all your facts right - you have got to have it clear in your mind. You cannot have it clear in your mind unless you have got that person's story. To suspend someone before you have even had a statement or even spoken to that person seems to be jumping the gun a bit. Again you are accountable for your decisions. It is OK communicating over the phone because that is not so important or writing letters... You have to weigh it up and think what is the most effective way and not how easy it is for you but the way in which you communicate with them and how it is going to effect that person.'

Although Tanya had no experience of acting as a supervisor, experience of poor supervision had enabled her to identify many of the key principles of effective supervision. It is crucial that the supervisor is fair, not only to the public and the service, but also to the midwife. The midwife needs to be given the opportunity of explaining what happened. When something apparently has gone wrong it is important to see the midwife in a 'face to face' interview. It is essential that the midwife is informed about exactly what she has done wrong and what alternative action the supervisor would have expected her to take given exactly the same set of circumstances. This information should be confirmed in writing. Communicating advice of suspension over the telephone enables the manager/supervisor to 'hide' from the full 'brunt' of the distress, anxiety and anger of the person to whom the information is communicated.

What was notable about this story is that the midwife did not think to look at the disciplinary policy to see whether it was being followed. The midwife's perception of the Industrial Relations Officer was that he had helped her. But although he had discussed the case with her in advance, he did not appear to have raised questions about the policy either. So that while he was well meaning and kind, it also raises questions about the level of training and knowledge of employment law that Industrial Relations Officers have. Under the Employment Protection Consolidation Act (1978) an employer must specify, in a contract of employment, any disciplinary rules applicable to the employee, or refer to a document which is reasonably accessible to the employee and which specifies such rules. It must also specify, by description or otherwise, a person to whom the employee can appeal if she is dissatisfied with any disciplinary decision relating to her, and a person to whom the employee can apply for the purpose of seeking redress of any grievance relating to her employment and the manner in which any such application should be made (Walton, 1990). The disciplinary procedure published by the Trust in 1993 stated that suspension was not considered to be disciplinary action, so a midwife could not appeal against it. It did, however, state that the reason for suspension must be confirmed in writing within seven days.

The operational maxim appeared to be suspend first and ask questions later and the Trust expected the supervisors to do this in order to protect 'the vulnerable public' and the reputation of the service. If the midwife was found 'not guilty' she could be reinstated and no harm was thought to befall her. This strategy, however, overlooked the enormous amount of psychological trauma that such a midwife experienced and the loss of confidence the midwife then had in the supervisors. This effected not only the individual midwife but radiated out and effected her colleagues generating low morale and a sense of 'always having to look over your shoulder' whilst practising. The Trust wanted anyone who was considered 'unsafe' to be suspended, but that raises questions about the criteria used to define unsafe practice, and exactly who determines the criteria.

Nancy who had experience of working as a supervisor spontaneously spoke of this incident and was able to shed further light on it. Nancy knew about this incident because she had discussed it with the supervisor who had suspended Tanya over the telephone. She described how supervision and management were confused resulting in poor support for the midwife. Note the very powerful use of metaphor which reflects the aggressive management approach of the Trust:

Nancy: '(Tanya) was actually suspended by a supervisor for allowing a woman to travel to Tarant in very early labour but she suddenly got on and delivered en route but because the papers got hold of it, the Trust had to be seen to be doing something so they suspended her pending investigation and in fact I do know the midwife - the manager at the time who had to suspend her did not really feel that it should be done but she was told by the Trust that she had to - otherwise it was her. So I am very uncomfortable with the power that the Trust has over the power of supervision, if you see what I mean.'

Researcher: 'Right, so what you are saying is that management and supervision functions have become confused?'

Nancy: 'I think they have been confused for a long time but it is becoming more confused now because they are - whereas before it was up to the individual manager - got her role confused - now we are bringing in a much higher level of management who want to be seen to be doing the right thing and it is - supervision has to be something that is totally outside that area. Outside that management area, it has to be - a supervisor needs to be someone not in any line of fire managerially at all.'

Confusion between supervision and management meant that the midwife was suspended as a 'face-saving exercise' for the Trust. Supervisors were hesitant to challenge senior management in case they were suspended. If the supervisor had challenged senior management would she have 'won the battle but lost the war?' In management it is so easy to restructure and lose people whose face does not fit. Should one stand up for one's principles at the risk of losing one's job? The additional conflict of being employer's advocate is well documented in the literature (Kirkham, 1995; Hughes, 1985). There appeared to be many parallels with the position the midwife found herself in with regard to her supervisor, and the position that the supervisor found herself in with regard to senior management. It is ironic that Tanya felt she was fortunate to have the Directorate manager present at her hearing when in fact it may have been that individual who had coerced the midwife manager against her better judgement to suspend the midwife.

The guidance issued by the Local Supervisory Authority states that it should be informed of any untoward incidents that the supervisor is investigating. The LSA should have supported the supervisor. It was unclear whether the LSA had been informed. Sadly even though the midwife had been completely cleared, a supervisor on a subsequent occasion had used this information to taunt her. Nancy pointed out:

'her supervisor has actually used it as a tool to mentally batter her and on a number of occasions... whenever she has questioned something that her manager/ supervisor says at a meeting it has been brought up, "Oh, you were suspended". So even though she was totally exonerated she has got that blight on her... that has been used as a tool to undermine... as a battering ram to intimidate her.'

Kargar (1993, p.22) expresses concern that there is no right of appeal for NHS midwives:

> 'Midwives being disciplined unfairly have to suffer gossip and innuendo in the work place. Their only chance to put their side of the case comes during official hearings, but by that time a great deal of damage has been done to their reputations.'

What is published by the local LSA is worthy of note; that supervisors have a duty to support midwives who act within their professional sphere of practice and common law.

The Midwives Autonomy Action Group, a group set up to publicize and fight unjustified midwife suspensions, has gone some way to addressing these issues. Beech (1993, p.44) states:

> 'An analysis of the experiences of independent midwives has revealed that a significant proportion of them have had disciplinary proceedings taken against them in recent years. Most of these proceedings were subsequently abandoned due to lack of supporting evidence... the power to suspend from practice is currently being abused. Even if a Supervisor thinks a midwife has committed an error of judgement or failed to adhere to the midwife's rules, it would have to be something very serious indeed to require suspension... if suspension is used without full justification it could result in successful legal action for damages by the midwife against the Supervisor and the Health Authority.'

Dimond (1994, p.23) provides another interesting perspective:

> 'If the supervisor of midwives is negligent in carrying out her duties as set out in the Rules, the Code of Practice and by the LSA... she may face professional conduct proceedings before the Professional Conduct Committee of the UKCC as being guilty of professional misconduct.'

Destructive use of power and oppression

Conflict between supervision and management was greatest when something had gone dramatically wrong. Midwives were unable to use the supervisor as a supporter because the management 'hat' took priority. When midwives needed support most - that is when something had gone radically wrong - they received it least. It was almost as though the rug had been pulled out from underneath them and left them floundering.

Karen described such an example of how supervisors were particularly powerful in oppression, that instead of supporting midwives they were disciplining them,

> Karen: 'I am just thinking about another case, which is not mine... she had a problem with a difficult delivery which went wrong and the supervisor and the manager of midwives wasn't at all supportive. She wouldn't say to her after the event, "Have a look at your notes, and see whether you need to add something", because sometimes you write things down in a hurry that you may want to add

a few things that are still fresh in your memory. She was not allowed that, she was not even allowed to look in her notes and I thought that was very unsupportive. She should have supported her to write really good notes and to amend the notes if she felt there wasn't everything she should write down about the particular case. It wasn't at all supportive. "You have not taken her temperature". She was not allowed to look at her notes, she could never see the notes, she was not given a copy, she could never defend herself.
Researcher: 'She wasn't even allowed a copy?'
Karen: 'No, no.'
Researcher: 'If she wrote the notes did she not own the record?'
Karen: 'Yes'
Researcher: 'Should she not be entitled to a copy?'
Karen: 'I think so, I think it should have been dealt with very differently.'

Although under normal circumstances there seemed to be a genuine will to support the midwife, when a delivery had gone wrong and the supervisor faced the threat of senior management involvement and the prospect of facing a legal claim of one to two million pounds for a brain damaged baby, a process of metamorphosis occurred in which the supervisor pulled the draw bridge up and left the midwife to drown in the moat. Poor support meant rather than assisting the midwife to write good records, access to records were prohibited. Karen's perceptions of supervisors was that they were in a very powerful position, there was no one to supervise the supervisors and they used their power destructively:

'If you don't do this, be careful you know, there will be a disciplinary action, it is definitely like that, it is what I find, I have experienced.'

Poor support to Karen meant threats of disciplinary action forced compliance. There appeared to be an implicit denial of choice. Karen appeared tired and sad and almost driven to inertia to avoid 'hassle'.

Control
The supervisor expected the midwives to contact them when anything untoward happened. She expected to be consulted and to direct operations. If midwives consulted the supervisor all was well but when midwives felt they knew what they were doing and used their own initiative they were severely punished - sometimes disciplined. It was almost as though the supervisor needed to be needed. Was this perhaps a sign of insecurity in herself or to justify the existence of her own job? She needed to be asked for her opinion and to feel in control. Providing the midwives contacted her and acknowledged this the supervisor supported them really well. Failing to acknowledge this carried severe penalties. The following case where the midwife 'got the discipline' illustrates the above points and is described by Fiona:

'one of them in particular was a case of taking a woman in the ambulance without medical support and the supervision then started after and not at the time, there was no supervision... the reason that she was disciplined was because she had not asked for supervision - she had not actually phoned and said "can

I speak to a supervisor, on a point of what shall I do in this situation?" She just decided this was an emergency and she must deal with it... the supervisor told her that had she phoned and discussed it with her, this supervisor would have supported her but she did not because she did it on her own.'

The midwife left and felt very bitter about what happened to her. The supervisor expected the midwife to abdicate 'ownership' of decision-making in relation to clinical problems to the supervisor and to become dependent on her. There was an implicit denial of choice/decision making. Lack of compliance was punished with disciplinary action.

Midwives cited examples of being treated like a child and being undervalued. One midwife recalled a very positive experience with a supervisor in another area for whom she had enormous respect:

'I would get what I call an adult response. You would have this one professional talking to another, it is not like a child talking to its mother... you want to feel that you are on a level with your supervisor... well I can remember actually for some reason telling Caroline (the supervisor) about the situation over the transferring the woman with PPH and before I finished... she jumped in like telling me what to do. I don't want to be told what to do, I am a professional in my own right.. I should not feel that I have to go into the "asking permission mode"'.

Poor support meant being told what to do and not being allowed to make one's own decisions. Poor support meant that ownership of the problem had shifted from the midwife to the supervisor. Supervisors need to exercise caution adopting a prescriptive approach like this because if the instructions issued do not effect a successful outcome, the supervisor can easily be blamed.

Supervisory interviews

Marion (a community midwife) felt that supervisors should treat a midwife 'as a human being and also as a grown-up'. The following description of a supervisory interview is interesting.

Marion: 'The first time I had to bring my equipment in to see that everything that was there was all in date and not out of date. That what was there was relevant and not everything and the kitchen sink... and then she asked to see all the books - you know - the Code of Conduct, Rules...'
Researcher: 'She wanted to see your copies?'
Marion: 'Yes, we had to take them. She had a form that she ticks them on.'
Researcher: 'How did you feel about that?'
Marion: 'Again I think that is very silly - why does she have to see what I have got? I mean it is up to me to make sure that when we get new copies from the UKCC you take the new one and you throw the old one in the bin. I feel that is when we are treated like little children.'

As Walton (1995) points out the practice of inspecting a midwife's bag which is part of the statutory framework 'does not seem congruous with the role of a midwife as an accountable practitioner. The idea certainly conflicts with the notion of the supervisor as a colleague and a peer'.

Marion described another supervisory interview with Mrs. Pope.

> Marion: 'Some supervisors - you go down there for ten minutes and the rest of your time - your allotted time - they talked about themselves and their problems which was not really what they were meant to do, I don't feel, not at that time anyway'
>
> Researcher: 'Can you give me an example of what you are talking about?'
>
> Marion: 'Yeah um - how awful it was for that person to be on her own and how awful it was when she left the place where she was working - the job was difficult and I can appreciate it was difficult but I don't think it was the right time for her to be talking about it.'

Poor support for Marion meant that the supervisor 'down-loaded' her own problems during supervisory interviews rather than focusing on the midwife and her professional practice needs. A role reversal had occurred: instead of the supervisor supporting the midwife, the supervisor was looking for support from the midwife.

Nancy described how her supervisory interview went:

> 'It was a waste of time… (I said) I feel quite happy with things the way they are because I did not feel that it was worth saying anything.'

Poor support for Nancy meant that she could not approach her supervisor with problems. Handy (1985) describes this as 'negative power'. He argues that all subordinates are, in a sense, gate-keepers to their supervisors, they screen out information and activities. The supervisor only sees what the midwife wants her to see. Negative power is the ability to filter or distort information. He argues:

> 'that negative power operates at times of low morale, irritation, stress, or frustration at the failure of other influence attempts... Successful, high morale organizations see little negative power. The use of negative power breeds lack of trust by the superior for the subordinate.'

A vicious cycle is created which reinforces each others behaviour. In a sense midwives operated 'underground', not identifying or discussing problems with their supervisors. So instead of discussing problems and smoothing things out at the first sign of trouble, because problems were 'hidden' they could never be adequately dealt with and they tended to escalate without the supervisor being aware that there was a problem.

Intimidation

Some midwives actually felt intimidated by supervisors:

> 'I can understand why midwives apparently do stupid things. I can understand that because you are continually bombarded and undermined and intimidated into actually feeling that you cannot actually make decisions. I have got the strength of what I was like before but I have seen midwives almost cracking.'

This intimidation however appeared to operate on two tiers as illustrated by Kate:

> 'I feel that she (the supervisor) is afraid of certain individuals and the supervisor prior to that was certainly intimidated by management - you have got to have a certain strength of character in order to carry out that kind of role and to be able to fight a few battles.'

The supervisors were not supported and they in turn did not support the midwives. The midwives did not support the supervisors.

Not being able to talk through feelings

Some of the midwives talked about not being able to talk through their feelings. One midwife talked about how angry and bitter midwives felt when supervisors failed to come and talk to them after a baby was found dead on a bed on a postnatal ward and they subsequently had to go to court. The mother of the baby had developed puerperal psychosis and although there was an open verdict it was believed she was instrumental in the baby's death. Fiona, a community midwife talked about a similar problem.

> 'One of the things I envy the Health Visitors is they actually have a separate group that they can go to with a counsellor of some kind who can talk through their feelings or their worries or their - without their being any - nothing is written down is taken anywhere else so it is never going to be used against them. I don't think that we get that type of support. I think you get burn out, I mean you get burn out at all levels but I think you tend to get something happening to midwives where they are hardening. You hear women say she was unkind from their perspective. I think that midwife has got a problem that she is not sympathising, empathising or able to give, she has probably given far more than she could cope with and has shut down... I think we need more help. I think in the past I have needed help but you do not feel you can say it because a midwife is seen as someone who is in charge... you take control and think control is a very good word, I think we do and you must not be out of control. I mean you are in control of that situation and in control of that woman in labour to a greater degree. Therefore you should be in control of yourself as well and if you are not, then you are not a good midwife.'

This recurring theme of 'control' is highly significant and appeared to operate at several levels. The midwife felt it was important to be 'in control' of herself and 'in control of that woman in labour'. The supervisor felt it was important to control the midwives. Senior management controlled the supervisor. This idea of control diffused and perpetuated through work at all levels within the maternity department within the Trust. No one was prepared to step out of line. Midwives were kept on a very tight rein. Control rather than support was the operational maxim. Although the supervisor's side of the story was not obtained, it is very apparent from talking to these midwives that midwives and supervisors seemed to see the aims of supervision very differently. The midwives perceived the supervisor's function as a controller whereas I believe the supervisors felt supervision was about ensuring the safety of mother and baby. Reflecting on Fiona's interview what struck me was the sudden awareness of the enormous amount of stress she worked under on a day to day basis in a deprived area in the community and the tremendous need for support and support groups in midwifery to provide the opportunity to talk through experiences and problems, rather than bottling them up inside. The long term effect of this made Fiona no longer able to respond adequately to the emotional needs of women because she simply could not cope any more.

Midwives were expected to stick to rigid protocols

Examples of rigid practices were given by several midwives. There was an expectation on behalf of supervisors that there was a single correct way of dealing with a problem and this was written down as a management policy. There was a management policy which stated that women delivering at home and who had a retained placenta, should be accompanied to hospital by a doctor. One midwife was disciplined for transferring a woman to hospital with a retained placenta in an ambulance without a medical escort. She had followed the GPs instructions and therefore had complied with the Midwives' Code of Practice. If the GP refused to attend, the supervisor expected the midwife to instruct the mother to use the yellow pages and find another GP. This perhaps reflects how far removed some supervisors have become from clinical practice. Delay in transferring the mother to hospital may put her at grave risk of post partum haemorrhage. A midwife can site an intravenous infusion, what additional skills would a GP be able to offer that a midwife did not have? Fiona discussed the problems she experienced with this particular protocol.

'I think on one occasion I have had to transfer someone from home into the maternity unit three miles away because she had... an unexpected undiagnosed pregnancy in her boyfriend's mother's house and the boyfriend's mother wanted her out. Now it was not going to make that situation better if I had hung on there any longer waiting for this third stage. It was getting aggressive - but practice - the policy - as far as my practice was concerned stated that I should not move that girl. Well I used my professional judgement - my judgement was as she was not bleeding and that we would be in an ambulance in which we would have better facilities than were in the house that was not very clean anyway, where I was liable to be clipped around the ear at any minute, that it was better that we moved the whole situation out but it was still wrong to have done it. I feel that when you get these statements coming out you need to say well no, but in this situation or that situation you might need to use your professional judgement. There isn't that - there is no flexibility. I think because the supervisor could not see at the time any situation from her practice where she had ever to contemplate having to move someone. She did not have the aggressive other adult there. I mean it is a one off but it is not flexible.'

Enforced compliance with rigid policies is a recipe for disaster in a rapidly changing maternity health scenario. Although policies can usefully serve as a tool for the inexperienced practitioner, there is a danger that the policy be viewed not as a tool and a guide but as a master - as Gordon (1984) argues 'an end in itself rather than a means to an end'. The policy will never be able to address the myriad of problems and challenges in the context in which the midwife is likely to face them. Midwives implementing the recommendations of the Expert Maternity Group need to work flexibly as they take on their own case loads. Rigid policies are likely to encourage mechanistic practice and stifle midwives working intuitively, they will restrict professional judgement and autonomy. Midwives may become bewildered and submerged by pages and pages of policies (which soon become outdated!). Rather than facilitating good practice the midwife becomes entrapped in the policy cobweb and ceases to think on her feet. Conformity and unquestioning slavish reliance on written policies as an 'ideal' characteristic in professional practice is obsolete and could jeopardize the safety of mother and baby.

The way ahead

No matter how well written the new Distance Learning pack is for the preparation of supervisors (ENB, 1992), it is the actual on site supervisor role model who will mould the trainee into a qualified supervisor. The trainee will acquire the knowledge that local supervisors use to interpret experience and generate social behaviour. Poor role models will produce poor supervisors. Education for existing supervisors as well as trainee supervisors is therefore crucial.

Schein (1988) states that allowing a client to become dependent on a consultant to find solutions to their problems, as comfortable as that might be for the consultant, is a prescription for failure in the helping process as far as complex human systems are involved. A parallel situation can be seen to be occurring between a midwife and her supervisor. The supervisor in this study felt comfortable making decisions for the midwives, it made her feel needed and important and justified her existence. If the midwife accepts expert advice, she may be able to solve her immediate problem but she may not be able to resolve a future problem. Encouraging dependence on another person to make professional decisions facilitates regression rather than progression of the midwife. Adopting the principles of process consultation as advocated by Schein (1988) may provide a more productive approach. Process consultation involves joint diagnosis of a problem. The supervisor should not attempt to solve the problem herself, instead she attempts to teach diagnostic and problem solving skills so that a midwife can manage organizational processes better herself and will be able to fix problems on a future occasion should they recur. The midwife should retain the diagnostic and remedial initiative. As such process consultancy is developmental in nature, it is psychologically difficult for a supervisor not to assume the expert role. When instructions from a supervisor are given however, they are often resented. A supervisor as a process consultant should endeavour to use questions. Schein (1988) argues that questions are in fact the more helpful intervention because it encourages and even forces the midwife to maintain the initiative. If the goal of process consultation is to help the midwife solve her own problems, to own the responsibility, then the question is the best way to communicate that expectation. So instead of using a didactic approach where the midwife is seen as an empty receptacle who needs to be filled with the knowledge and wisdom that emanates from the supervisor, Socratic approaches actually encourage the human process of learning. The supervisor could respond to the midwife's questions with further questions, so that the onus is always on the midwife to formulate an action plan. This is important because at the end of the day the supervisor is not actually there in the immediate clinical situation and may not appreciate all the factors involved and furthermore the midwife is accountable for her actions. As such a reflective style of learning is created. This process style of learning becomes particularly relevant in a modern society where midwifery in undergoing a rapid period of metamorphosis. As Schon (1990) points out:

'In the swampy lowland, messy confusing problems defy technical solutions. The irony of the situation is that the problems on the high ground tend to be relatively unimportant to individuals or society at large, however great their technical interest may be, while in the swamp lie the problems of greatest human concern.'

Fiona, grappling with the problem of a mother with a retained placenta at home with aggressive relatives and no flying squad is a very good example of this.

Supervisors need to produce an environment of psychological safety where problems can be safely aired. It is important to avoid personal humiliation and loss of face or self-esteem. If a pre-requisite for a supervisor was to have advanced professional education, for example a diploma or a degree specifically in midwifery, this may go some way to help rational decisions being made. Counselling skills would also be advantageous. Advanced professional education alone, however, will not be enough to correct such a political mess where the supervisors themselves feel so threatened. Supervisors need assertiveness training and support mechanisms. Whilst it is recognized that, in some situations, suspension is called for because it has such a devastating effect on the midwife, perhaps one way forward would be to suspend a midwife from duty only if two or more senior supervisors in two different Trusts think that it is appropriate. During preparation for the role of a supervisor it may be worth exploring with the trainee how they would feel if they were suspended themselves. An independent appeals mechanism needs to be set up. Clinical management policies should be completely phased out and supervisors should encourage midwives to apply the principles in 'The Scope for Professional Practice' (UKCC, 1992).

Purposive sampling may have attracted a small unhappy minority of midwives who wanted to talk about bad experiences. However an alternative argument may be that a lot of midwives who had been suspended may be embarrassed by that fact and rather than wanting to talk about it may prefer to conceal it. Most midwives in my opinion have felt that it is mainly independent midwives who have faced gross injustices at the hands of supervisors. This research tells a sad and different story. I hope this will be read by midwives training to be supervisors, as a result I hope they will reflect on the impact that their actions have on their colleagues and that they will make supervision a tool of empowerment and support rather than one of oppression.

Acknowledgements

I would like to acknowledge the constant support and encouragement of my research supervisor Val Levy who empowered me to successfully complete this research.

I would like to acknowledge the help of all the midwives who contributed to this research project and who taught me what supervision meant to them.

References

Beech, L.B. (1993). 'Supervision of midwives' *AIMS Journal* Vol. 5, No. 2, Summer pp.1-3.

Chalmers, I., Enkin, M., Keirse, M.J.N.C. (1989). *Effective Care in Pregnancy and Childbirth.* Oxford: Oxford University Press.

Dimond, B. (1994). *The Legal Aspects of Midwifery.* Hale: Books for Midwives Press.

English National Board (1992). *Preparation of Supervisors of Midwives An open learning programme Module 3 The role and the responsibility of the supervisor in dealing with alleged professional misconduct.* London: English National Board.

Enkin, M., Keirse, M.J.N.C., Renfrew, M.J., Neilson, J.P. (1995). *Pregnancy and Childbirth Module The Cochrane Pregnancy and Childbirth Database (database on disk and CDROM) The Cochrane Collaboration Issue 2 Oxford Update Software* Available from B.M.J. Publishing Group. London.

Field, P.A., Morse, J.M. (1985). *Nursing Research. The Application of Qualitative Approaches.* London: Chapman and Hall.

Gordon, R.D. (1984). 'Research application: identifying the use and misuse of formal models in nursing practice' in Benner, P. (Ed). *From Novice to Expert Excellence and Power in Clinical Nursing Practice.* California: Addison-Wesley Publishing Company.

Handy, C. (1985). *Understanding Organisations* (Third Edition) Harmondsworth: Penguin.

Hughes, D. (1985). 'Supervisors of midwives' *Midwives Chronicle and Nursing Notes.* Vol. 98, No. 1174, Nov p.299.

Kargar, I. (1993). 'Whither supervision?' in *Nursing Times* October 6, Vol. 89, No. 40, p.22.

Kirkham, M. (1995). 'The history of midwifery supervision' in ARM (Ed). *Super-Vision Consensus Conference Proceedings.* Hale: Books for Midwives Press.

Lincoln, Y., Guba, E. (1985). *Naturalistic Enquiry.* Beverley Hills, California: Sage Publications.

Ministry of Health (1937). *Supervision of Midwives Circular 1620* Ministry of Health

National Health Service Management Executive (1993). *A Vision for the Future - The Nursing, Midwifery and Health Visiting Contributions to Health and Health Care.* London: Department of Health.

Schein, E.H. (1988). *Process Consultation Vol 1 Its Role in Organisational Development.* Reading, Massachusetts: Addison - Wesley Publishing Company.

Schon, D. (1990). *Educating the Reflective Practitioner.* San Francisco: Jossey Bass.

Simms, C., McHaffie, H., Renfrew, M.J., Ashurst, H. (1994). *A Midwifery Research Database MIRIAD* Hale: Books for Midwives.

Spradley, J. (1979). *The Ethnographic Interview.* New York: Holt, Rinehart and Winston.

UKCC (1992). *The Scope of Professional Practice.* London: UKCC.

UKCC (1994). *The Midwives Code of Practice.* London: UKCC.

Walton, F. (1990). *Encyclopaedia of Employment Law and Practice.* London: Professional Publishing.

Walton, I. (1995). 'Conflicts in supervision of midwives' in ARM (Ed). *Super-Vision Consensus Conference Proceedings.* Hale: Books for Midwives.

CHAPTER THIRTEEN

Independent Midwives' Views of Supervision

Jill Demilew
is Quality Assurances Manager (Midwifery) at Tower Hamlets Healthcare Trust, London. She has been a midwife for 18 years and has worked within and alongside the NHS, including 8 years as an independent midwife. She was a founder member of South East London Midwifery Group Practice (one of the first to contract their service into the NHS). In 1995, she moved back into direct NHS employment within a unique midwifery structure to facilitate an autonomous accountable service in a devolved organizational model.

Introduction

During 1991, I had been practising as an 'independent midwife' for the previous three years and nearing the end of postgraduate studies at the University of the South Bank London. I trained as a midwife in the late 1970s when the biomedical model was the dominant paradigm in the provision of the British maternity services. It enshrined childbirth in a 'mechanistic' vision to be controlled and managed, underpinned with the promise of increased safety for mother and child.

The organization of the maternity services was hierarchical and controlled by one profession, medicine, and centred in hospitals. Midwifery practice had become organized in a hospital based nursing model and professional practice was expected, by many, to mirror the beliefs and practices of our medical colleagues.

During the 1980s the intraprofessional and interprofessional tensions within midwifery practice and the maternity services were becoming evident. Women and midwives began to evaluate the service and critique some effects of this particular organization of care. Robinson (1985a, 1985b) undertook large scale surveys of midwifery practice which demonstrated the erosion of the role of midwives and a subsequent deskilling within professional practice. She also noted that the use of professional resources within this system was wasteful because of the duplication of work by midwives and doctors.

Women who used the service were requesting a more personalized service and one in which being given better information enabled them to make their own choices (Graham and McKee, 1979; Garcia, 1982; Reid and McIlwaine, 1980; Oakley, 1979; Cartwright, 1979; Reid, 1986).

Tensions were becoming more apparent within the relationship of midwifery practice to nursing practice. This was highlighted during the application of a new financial reward structure in nursing and midwifery in 1988 namely 'Clinical Grading Structure'. The application of this structure in midwifery was very incoherent and dependent on geographical and employment location rather than actual professional practice. Midwives had wanted a separate salary structure in recognition that midwifery is a different practice from nursing practice. Midwives have a minority numerical status in the United Kingdom Central Council for Nursing Midwifery and Health Visiting (UKCC), a single statutory governing body formed in 1983. Decision making by midwives for professional practice could be outvoted by virtue of sheer 'numbers' at Council level. This organizational structure continued the pattern of lack of control over professional practice, which mirrored the loss of control of professional practice through structural organization of hospitals, where midwifery was subsumed within the nursing hierarchy.

This is the background in which I chose to study 'independent midwives'. It was a sociological analysis of a 'crisis' within the midwifery profession. The focus is in the fact that midwives are legislated to be autonomous practitioners but in the 1991 organization of maternity services they had little more than semi-professional status. Role erosion had resulted in problems with recruitment and retention (Fern, 1991) and intraprofessional tensions (Flint, 1985; Warren, 1988; Weitz, 1987).

Independent midwives were those midwives who elected to practice outside the employment of the NHS Maternity Services. They were a small growing minority who represented change in the social organization of care provision for birthing women and their families (41 out of 32,000 practising midwives). They were then part of the leading edge of a destabilized system of maternity services, who by their presence presented a viable alternative model of care and practice organization. They represented part of the challenge to the then organization of midwifery and maternity services.

Supervision of midwifery practice and the research

The main themes of the research looked at 'relationships'. The relationship of midwife to herself, midwife to woman, midwife to midwife colleagues, midwife to supervisor, midwife to medical colleagues and midwife to other professional colleagues.

The practice of supervision of midwifery became a central issue during my research. Its very presence in the structure of professional practice and the ways in which it was then practised had the potential to affect service provision in an enabling or obstructive way. This became particularly apparent when considering access to services and facilitating excellent quality services to birthing women and their families. The following account will concentrate on those findings in my research which are pertinent to supervision of midwifery. Finally, I will discuss the implications of the findings to the changing organization of midwifery and maternity services today.

The research

There is a tension in British midwifery between the legislated right to practice as a practitioner in ones own professional role and the actual practice of midwives in the NHS organization, in which they are restricted from realizing their full role. Starting with this general observation I wanted women practising as midwives in a specific context to express their professional practice from their perspective. My motivation was to gain an understanding and information about independent midwifery practice, in a systematic way. I had two hypotheses. Firstly, that in the context of this central tension, a group of practitioners who realize their practice as autonomous professionals may experience more frequent attempts at being controlled by professional and organizational mechanisms. Secondly, that during any time of change in organization or belief systems of professionals and consumers, any mechanisms of control will become clearly obvious. Any information gained had the potential to help towards changing midwifery practice and the organization of maternity services for the benefit of women as mothers, their families and midwives as practitioners.

Independent midwives were chosen because they are self employed. The mechanism of controlling their practice is not by managerial jurisdiction but via the professional supervisory mechanism required by statute. During 1991, 41 midwives had notified their intention to practice as 'independent midwives'. The majority were members of two organizations, Independent Midwives Association (IMA) and the Northern Independent Midwives Association (NIMA). There were 53 members of whom 43 were listed as practising full time. I contacted all full time members since the other members were associate status and just starting practice. I eventually interviewed 32 midwives who were representative of those practising throughout England which was important to see if there was any regional variation of their experiences. The sample covered 78 per cent of midwives practising independently.

This research was designed as an in-depth qualitative study which had three parts. A comprehensive literature review was completed. A documentary analysis was undertaken on all material from the review, concentrating on the key concepts of supervision, practitioner, accountability and legislation. The final part was undertaking informal semi-structured individual interviews concentrating on four areas. These were exploring individuals ideas about professional practice, their knowledge, experiences and views of supervision of midwifery, factors enabling or obstructing their professional practice and finally what their vision was of the future of midwifery practice in Britain.

The interviews took place over an eleven week period. They varied between one and a half to four hours each. They were recorded in longhand and then entered on a word processor. The data was categorized as themes and patterns emerged which I compared with sociological theoretical contexts. Finally the findings suggested some insights which have implications for the midwifery profession, the maternity services, women and their families.

Research findings

Social profile

The midwives were mature women with an average age of 37 years. Over two thirds had dependent children. One third had children under school age. The majority were experienced practitioners, the average length of practice being almost nine years. There was a wide range in length of NHS practice before changing to self employed practice varying from 0 to 33 years. Half of the midwives changed within ten years of qualifying. Nearly two thirds are graduates or were currently undergraduates. The majority are registered nurses but two registered via the 'direct entry' route. Half of the midwives had specific interests in women's health issues including those who had worked in teaching (Midwifery and Family Planning, 2), worked in primary care in 'developing' countries (five) and as National Childbirth Trust Teachers (six, five of them before they were midwives). When leaving the security of NHS employment, half were solvent and able to accept the financial risk whilst the others used government Enterprise Allowance Schemes ensuring a weekly income for a year. Others took bank loans to pay for a reliable car and equipment. Most went into partnership working with a colleague who shared a similar philosophy of practice.

The midwives reflect women in the general population in that some have dependants and marked family responsibilities. They show it is possible to practice in this way with or without substantial family commitments. There was a noticeable pattern of newer independent midwives to transfer from employed to independent practice sooner after qualification. The life experiences of many of these women enabled them to see birth outside of the institution. They had had the opportunity to view childbirth as non medicalized, pro women, family and community. This lends itself to its own philosophy of childbirth in which women are seen as healthy and birth is a normal process. They had the ability to question their practice and how it affects themselves, women and families. They were unlikely to fit easily in a hierarchical system in which midwives realized their practice in a nursing organizational model.

Reasons to practice

The midwives stated many different reasons for choosing to enter midwifery varying from personal experiences of birth, personal philosophy, a route to professional development and complete pragmatism. For example:

> 'I returned to midwifery (after a long break) because I kept seeing friends have bad experiences in births and thought what's wrong? I had two wonderful homebirths myself.'

> 'after nursing became very politicised during a course 'The Political Economy of Health' at night school... it changed my life. I already had a place to train as a midwife so went... the whole system was geared to doctors, not to women or midwives... not represent home and happiness but ego and high-powered stuff. I wonder whether I'd have noticed it had I not done that course, none of the other student midwives noticed it.'

> 'I did midwifery for another qualification, I didn't particularly like obstetrics, seemed terrifyingly out of my depth.'

However they all had the same three reasons for entering 'independent practice' which were:

- To practice as a midwife as an autonomous practitioner
- To be able to give continuity of care to women and enable homebirth
- To practice in accordance with their philosophy of birth.

For example:

'angry over other midwives rudeness, unreasonable policies, didn't look at women as individuals. Doctors taking over or midwives letting them especially in normal cases, also in terms, when women went over the bounds of normal instead of allowing options they were told what had to happen.'

'as evidence emerged re the safety of homebirth and desirability of DOMINO scheme we couldn't offer it because we did not have the time to do it, to listen, and I not want to end my practice like that' (previous community midwife)

'... have an overwhelming faith in women's ability to deliver. To go and cherish people you need touch and massage, not pethidine and hard beds... people couldn't cope with that in hospital, being a topic of conversation... people eventually realized what I did benefited women.'

The nature of professional practice

The changes in these independent midwives' organization of practice and their professional practice challenges the sociological theories of professions and professionalization. Instead of seeking an increase in professional status through increasing their professional authority over women or distancing themselves from women, they perceived themselves as being jointly responsible with the woman and of being closer to women, 'with woman' sharing maximum information. They do, however, adhere to other ideas of professionalism in that they zealously claim specialized knowledge, the right to clinical decision making and making clinical judgements. They have specialized training and submit to an ethical code developed and policed by the profession.

Perhaps one of the most interesting findings was that the midwives observed a change in their practice. This was in the direction of the women who had an increase in responsibility and power, the more autonomously these midwives practised. As the midwives changed their previously semi-professional organization of practice into autonomous professional practice, it increased the power of the women who they served. For example:

'quite difficult because I have changed the way I work. In the community in NHS, at the beginning I used to take quite a lot of responsibility myself. Even though NHS is a service where a woman can decide what she will do, as an independent midwife you're clearer on the fact, that is what happens. Don't have to tell what she ought to do re NHS policies, thus it is far freer.'

'initially felt it was completely me, when things happened. In retrospect, not significant, just happened e.g. transfer to hospital for caesarean or forceps delivery. I felt guilty, terrible, stressful then with more experience moved a zillion miles from that, now… what will happen will happen, she'll give as much as she can, I'll give it everything I've got… time, love, one to one care, encouragement, give her sound decision making information and discuss it through. My responsibility is to empower them to feel they've done all they can therefore whatever they've done is a success.'

The organization of midwifery care and the philosophy of birth which midwives hold affects the professional relationship and way in which one practices professionally. These midwives defined the role of a midwife as having several functions. Usually each midwife defined her role as having many functions. The most frequently mentioned was that of an advocate to empower women (77 per cent). About half of them specified that they were specialists in normal childbirth and educators, a knowledge resource for women (45 per cent). Over a third directly saw their role as encompassing being political in which a responsibility lay in recognizing the social implications for women, midwives and society concerning issues surrounding pregnancy and childbirth (39 per cent). Nearly a quarter saw part of their role as being a counsellor and friend. Below are some examples of their insights,

'one of the biggest things is to empower women, enable them to make informed choices: in hospital felt knowledge was guarded, less knowledge shared is more power to the practitioner, creates more barriers is intimidating: the barrier doesn't make for good outcomes in terms of clients wishes. It's different now.' (advocacy)

'to provide her with a safety net, ensure parameters of safety are made clear to her… monitor within the parameters of safety, my expertise is there, which women do not usually have.' (expert in the normal)

'resource, lots of information, an education resource re pregnancy, breastfeeding etc.' (educator)

'have a very special relationship with women: long term consequences with bonding and breastfeeding… yet that will be in the next generation… so important; like an invisible effect, lots is invisible, the prevention of problems is invisible and difficult to quantify. That I feel is my biggest contribution. The unquantifiable: the quality of relationships between parent and child.' (political)

'befriend a woman for a time in life when you need a friend with the knowledge they don't have… friendship is important to enable women to be themselves during labour and early parenting: not want barriers at those times.' (friendship, counsellor)

The last area of professional practice which I explored considered where the midwife would seek support in the event of any conflict being present between themselves and a woman. Nearly a third (31 per cent) said they had never been in this situation.

However, those who had been uncomfortable professionally with a woman's decision making did seek to resolve this. Many sought support in several areas. The most frequent step was to share knowledge with the woman (87 per cent). Most accessed advice from other professional colleagues, other midwives, supervisors of midwives and obstetricians. Eleven midwives specifically mentioned supervisors of midwives (35 per cent). They reported mixed responses in their experience of supervision in these circumstances. It seemed either the supervisors were superb, or they were obstructive. Only three midwives viewed this support as positive. For example:

> 'supervisor was brilliant, had lots of problems in the past with this woman, knew her from her last birth, she'd been labelled. She lent me two hospital entonox cylinders, gave me narcan,... this woman lived out on the moors... if this woman has a problem, we'll use the helicopter if it snows.'

> 'the supervisors aren't putting women's interests first at all. Because these women didn't conform to hospital policies and wanted continuity of carer they end up at home in situations where I don't always feel is in their best interest. If acknowledge women are at risk, they should do anything to get them in. If all policies are not followed that's less important (re not being given an honorary contract in a Health Authority where women want continuity of care from a midwife with whom they have established trust).'

Central to all the midwives was that they would stay with the woman's choice. They saw this as the cornerstone of professional practice, of establishing trust between themselves and the woman. Equally this trust included access to all sources of knowledge i.e. research evidence and consultations with Consultant Obstetricians or other specialists. The following findings explore in depth the particular relationship of supervision to midwifery practice in the 'independent model' of practice.

Independent midwifery practice model and relationship with supervision

Supervision is a professional activity. The Local Supervising Authority (LSA, previously Regional Heath Authorities) requires supervision to be carried out by a practising midwife. The main focus is 'protection' of the public by enabling excellent quality midwifery care to all women. Midwives who became supervisors before 1990 were usually senior managers (UKCC, Isherwood 1988).

They also have loyalties to the organization for whom they work as well as to midwives and mothers for whom they are to be advocates. Fern (1991) comments on this structural position and reflects that is a facet of semi-professional status. She states,

> 'The senior semi-professional becomes concerned with maintaining and representing the organization, rather than leading the profession.'

The relationship between the supervisory and managerial role has been and continues to be widely debated. In theory the supervisor is expected to exercise these roles independently and judiciously. There has been an observed difference between theory and practice. The actual conflict of the dual roles is amply explored by Hughes (1985), Flint (1985), Warren (1988) and Isherwood (1988). However, Lansdell (1989) perceives this duality as having great potential since to resolve professional supervisory issues, one almost always requires managerial action.

The supervisory function has potential power especially concerning professional regulation and control of practice. It is the main professional disciplinary tool. During the late 1980s, one of the central questions concerning midwifery practice was in whose interest supervision was being exercised? This was placed firmly on the agenda through several cases publicized in the national media. They were Jilly Rosser who was removed from the professional register then reinstated (Editorial MIDIRS, 1988); Chris Warren, a community midwife suspended for delivering a woman at a planned homebirth before the arrival of the second midwife (Cronk, 1988) and Mary Cronk, a community midwife who refused to obey local health authority policy if she professionally judged it to be not in a clients' interests (Flint, 1987).

Martin (1990), from an in-depth study of midwifery professional conduct cases, concluded that midwives are in effect damned if they do and damned if they don't. Her analysis showed that midwives were disciplined for not exercising accountability if they followed local policies or medical instructions blindly and disciplined for exercising professional clinical judgement and not following local policies. The inherent conflict in the structure and organization of midwifery practice is *that the midwife may be seen to be the controller (practitioner) and the controlled (semi-professional status)*. Independent midwifery organization of practice may indicate some of the implications different organizational models could have for professional practice. Midwife activist groups organized study days to analyse the course and implications of regulation of their profession (Hughes, 1986). The Midwives Action and Autonomy Group (MAAG) formed in 1988 to fight what was perceived as increasing restrictions on rights of practitioners because seven out of thirty independent midwives were suspended or under investigation by the UKCC (Flint, 1987). It has been interpreted by some observers as intraprofessional conflict between those midwives who exercised their rights to practice and some midwives exercising the supervisory mechanism to discipline these midwives punitively (Flint, 1985; Hughes, 1985; Warren, 1988; Cronk, 1988; Briggs, 1989; Flint, 1987; Editorial MIDIRS, 1988).

Knowledge of supervision

Only five of the thirty one midwives acknowledged that their education about supervision had been informative and comprehensive. All five were the most recently qualified and had trained during a time when the cases of Jilly Rosser, Chris Warren and Mary Cronk were in the national media. All of them had midwifery tutors who were active members of the Association of Radical Midwives. Their education included discussion of the role and potential conflicts within supervision. Six midwives were unable to remember any education regarding supervision. The majority (77 per cent) said that what they had was insufficient for actual practice in that it was brief, cursory and not meaningfully taught.

For example:

> 'one lecture as a student and an in-service training session. The Director of Midwives gave a talk about supervision. It was a one dimensional linear thing, a hierarchical diagram: no-one communicated what it really meant in reality. Always got the impression no-one really knew what a supervisor did do, more a disciplinary, a hierarchical place to discipline midwives.'

Experience of supervision whilst an NHS employee

Nearly two thirds of the midwives were unaware of supervision for themselves (61 per cent).

> 'until became an independent midwife never knew what the supervisor was at all, it wasn't important, you worked for the hospital.'

However more than half were aware of supervision of colleagues in their unit or nationally (55 per cent). All were seen as negative experiences for the midwives and midwifery practice.

> 'a midwife on "nights" who was put into a white coat, taken out of her Sisters' navy blue uniform to distinguish her from anyone else. It was talked about as the role of the supervisor being paramount.'

> 'my whole training was coloured by the Jilly Rosser case, as a student I also attended the trial, took my children to support her and it has definitely affected the way I practice. Being at the trial affected me deeply seeing the unjust methods used and the way they treated Jilly, the callousness. I didn't know Jilly. At the time I found it impossible to believe that midwives could treat each other in this way.'

Eighteen supervisory episodes were reported of which nearly threequarters were perceived as unhelpful, negative or destructive. A quarter did find the experience helpful supportive and enabling.

Examples of good support were:

> 'I went voluntarily to my supervisor when a woman committed suicide with psychosis, very good regarding my grieving.'

> 'where supervisors were tutors not managers, it was different, could relate to them, not so afraid of what they might do, because really nice people and knew that they were very supportive of midwives.'

Examples of unhelpful support were:

> 'had a final interview for a community midwifery post: a few days later I made a drug error on a very busy postnatal ward (it was prescribed in the wrong

dosage by the doctor, an analgesic). The supervisor said, in this case she would proceed immediately to a final warning. I had to have supervised practice, which meant not being able to 'hold' the ward drug keys or make any kind of decisions. A vague feeling I had been dishonest... this was very painful when previously I was used to making decisions. At the end she asked me twice whether I had learned or benefited. When I replied "No" she nearly killed me. The supervisor said that I wasn't fit to practice so it dragged on, no decision and six months became a year. I wouldn't "kiss the rod". In the end, let the question of whether I was suitably chastened drop, since I was so stubborn about it. I was given a temporary contract then a permanent contract, finally a community post. I knew other people were in the same predicament as me, in the hospital... but never spoke about it, our eyes just met occasionally. One of the worst things was the secrecy; it allowed gossip to flourish, the whispering.'

Experience of investigatory supervisory episodes as an independent midwife

These ranged from informal interviews and counselling to formal investigatory mechanisms.

Two thirds of the midwives had been through an investigatory process (20 midwives). A quarter of the midwives had been investigated more than once. In fact, five had been investigated on three separate occasions.

Thirty two separate incidents were reported. All of them were instigated by supervisors a minority of which were following requests or complaints by other professionals (6). Four of these were from junior medical staff (Senior House Officer) and midwives.

A quarter of the midwives had formal disciplinary investigations at the Local Supervising Authority. All needed professional and legal advice using the services of the Royal College of Midwives. Solicitors were consulted officially and unofficially. Brian Raymond who acted on behalf of Jilly Rosser and Wendy Savage in their professional conduct cases, was consulted in seven out of the eight cases. The outcome was that two of the midwives were suspended from practice for different periods of time pending investigation and were reinstated to 'supervised practice'.

An analysis of the investigations, which were explored at length during interview, revealed that half concerned differences in clinical practice and clinical decision making as measured by local policies. One in five were appropriate retrospective enquiries reviewing adverse pregnancy outcomes i.e. intrauterine or neonatal death or babies who were initially ill. However, what caused the greatest concern was the process of supervision. The midwives were heavily critical in that the investigations were experienced as being unsupportive, punitive and rather negative. They saw that there was a demonstrable lack of trust by the supervisor of the midwife. The process often seemed to be one of blame-labelling until proven otherwise.

Examples are shown opposite.

'disagreement with management of a woman who had ruptured membranes at term for over twenty four hours. The current policy was to induce labour after this time. However, research suggests that this does not need to happen and that a woman has more options than this which would not increase the risk to her or her baby. The midwife was called to account for not following a particular medical management model despite having discussed the research and options with the woman.'

'A retrospective enquiry following a neonatal death of a baby aged two days. The review of care by the local supervisor was thorough and demonstrated evidence of good midwifery practice. She was very supportive to the midwife involved. The baby had been reviewed by the General Practitioner and a Paediatric Registrar prior to his death. Post mortem revealed that the death was inevitable due to damage to pulmonary tissue from an infection probably occurring in the second trimester. The resultant damage was incompatible with supporting extrauterine life, the baby succumbing to congestive cardiac failure. The Local Supervising Authority started a formal enquiry process seven months following the baby's' death. In the interim there was no communication through the supervisory mechanism of any concerns regarding the midwife's practice. The supervisory outcome ended in a meeting of the midwife with the Regional Nurse and the Regional Solicitor. They apologized to the midwife and acknowledged that she had practised entirely appropriately. This was, however, at great emotional cost to the midwife having to consult with a solicitor, making statements, involving the parents at a time of their grieving and in a time frame which was very lengthy over several months.'

The midwives shared several instances of supervision which suggested that the supervisor needed to show a degree of control of the midwife. For example:

'a midwife was summonsed to see a supervisor because a consultant complained that the midwife hadn't kept any clinical casenotes on a woman who had needed transfer to hospital for some care postnatally. The woman had her casenotes with her all the time and the midwife had shared these with the medical team at the time of transfer.'

'a midwife was summonsed to the supervisor following a transfer of a woman to hospital because a breech presentation was diagnosed during labour. She was asked to make a statement, even though her colleague had cared for that woman during labour, not herself.'

Independent midwives view of supervision through experience

Sadly only two midwives commented that they had positive experiences. Both of them also commented adversely regarding the bureaucracy and hierarchy which could be obstructive. Comments were:

'on the whole apart from one supervisor (overly stroppy), they've been friendly, reasonably approachable until comes to a potentially difficult clinical situation re clinical judgement.'

'supervisors 'x' and 'y' you could feel easy informing them of every client. This was particularly when there were situations bordering on a deviation from normal as well as obvious deviation. I knew we were able to get advice and support and they were not going to interfere but offered and opened all the facilities i.e. day unit, scanning, obstetric consultation... anything which was in the best interests of the client. This seems the way it should be going, discuss anything without being censured for it.'

The rest of the midwives expressed their view of supervision as being non existent and useless (33 per cent ten midwives) or obstructive in which the supervisor had different beliefs from their own (55 per cent seventeen midwives). Supervision was understandably also affected according to individual personalities and relative clinical experience (40 per cent twelve midwives). Examples were:

'no use to me at all at the moment, it feels as if I'm supporting the supervisor and trying to get things out of her, it's like playing games... I like clarity.' (useless)

'lots of supervision seems to be from a defensive position, all out to catch you out, find any little mistake and make it into a mountain or try to find out every case so they can work out how they can manage it i.e. impose their own rules on you which are not necessarily research based or a woman's choice.' (controlling)

'it seems to be a matter of different personalities, can't be just a matter of hospital policies or wouldn't be so different from one supervisor to another in the same unit... different styles and interpretation of supervisors role.' (individual difference)

Some core attributes emerged which defined a supervisor. A good enabling supervisor was someone who shared a similar philosophy of birth and midwifery practice and was actively supportive of women and midwives. A poor supervisor was characterized as someone who tried to control the midwife through hostile interviews, blocking access to investigations and consultations, was out of date regarding midwifery knowledge and was primarily doctor advocate rather than midwife or woman advocate.

Strategies adopted by midwives and supervisors in their relationships

Midwives

The midwives were all clear that their prime aim was to facilitate women's access to the best quality care available according to individual needs. The following strategies evolved which proved to help the midwife-supervisor relationship. If a midwife was working in several health districts, it was helpful to arrange for one supervisor to check equipment and then write a letter stating this had taken place which could be acceptable to all the other supervisors. Some midwives invited a supervisor to meet them in their working premises to promote the mutuality of the relationship and have an expectation of friendly professional advice. Some midwives discovered that the supervisory relationship could change through initial conflict. Through demonstrating professional knowledge and sharing clinical decision making, there is a route towards mutual professional respect. Some midwives either notified each client to a supervisor in good faith that they will help if it is needed, whilst other midwives stopped notifying each client to stop any attempted exercise of management or control over the midwife's practice.

Strategies adopted by some supervisors in the relationship to independent midwives

The norm was to marginalize the midwives by not including their expertise in policy formation where it directly affects their practice. They never consulted these midwives when compiling prescriptive 'lists' of equipment which the midwives were expected to have for 'safe' practice.

They were further marginalized in circumstances in which they were accepted to practice in hospital when employed as bank or agency midwives but when they needed to continue caring for a client in the hospital following a transfer, they were not enabled to do so through issuing an honorary contract or terms of access' document. Thankfully some supervisors fought very hard in their organizations to enable this continuity of midwifery care. They did so on the woman's behalf acknowledging her choice and needs.

Some of the midwives acknowledged the difficulty of supervisors in the organization of maternity services. For example:

> 'if they are a good supervisor, they're so tired of beating their heads against brick walls: no sense of achievement for them. What's in it for them, in a punitive, hierarchical system where there's lots of opportunities to crack heads but little chance to give praise where praise is due.'

Summary of the supervisory relationship

The midwives clearly and powerfully articulated supervision as being usually practised in a controlling obstructive way. The irony is that it often had the effect of obstructing their clients from accessing the best quality care. This is the very opposite intention of supervision. Here is a practice situation in which midwives are committed to providing excellent quality care and by implication 'safest' care and yet the professional mechanism which is meant to be the cornerstone of providing a 'safe' service for women was itself obstructing this happening. There were thankfully some notable exceptions which provided the route to identifying qualities of excellent supervision. *Poor supervision* was identified as more likely to take place in three particular sets of circumstances. Firstly, when there were identifiable differences between the midwife and the supervisor in their respective ideas about pregnancy, birth and the place of these in society. Secondly, the midwife and supervisor may have very different ideas about the nature of professional practice in general and midwifery practice in particular. Thirdly, the last tension would occur when there was a difference in knowledge, understanding and expectations of the role of a supervisor and of supervision itself.

The future of supervision

Independent midwives were clear in their view of how supervision should be practised to protect the public and facilitate autonomous professional practice through enabling the provision of excellent quality midwifery services. One third, who were very experienced clinically and politically aware, thought it inappropriate to have supervision at all in its current format. On reflection, having worked with many supervisors in the English Health Authorities, they felt that there must be better and different mechanisms to reach the same goal.

> 'it's a double bind, very nice to have a guide and counsellor to whom you can turn to discuss matters, although other independent midwives fit this role for me more satisfactorily than the supervisor, because supervisors on the whole do not have any concept of how we work, they're on a different wavelength… has become a policing role which predominates therefore is demoralising and degrading for us as professionals. Other professionals don't have policing agents in the same way. It's a confusing system, one person having the dual role of police and support: it is a practical impossibility.'

Three positive functions of supervision were identified. Supervision should function as an advocacy mechanism for women and midwifery practice (75 per cent, 23 midwives). Secondly, supervision played a mediatory role in enabling a midwife to access laboratory facilities, investigations, consultations and to continue midwifery care for women in the hospital setting (33 per cent, ten midwives). Finally that there is the potential for a midwife to have a supervisory relationship and that this should be with one supervisor (25 per cent, eight midwives).

The independent midwife and the NHS

In 1991 midwives did not have any right of access to pathology services, ultrasound screening, direct referral to obstetricians or other specialities as practising midwives. In many maternity services, midwives would sign requests for laboratory investigations but this was usually done to streamline service provision rather than acknowledging that midwifery practice should encompass use of laboratory and investigatory facilities. The woman had the right of access to all these services free of charge.

The independent midwives shared their experiences of negotiating with professional colleagues in the NHS. These professionals were representative across the maternity services and included obstetricians, GPs, social workers, paediatricians, health visitors and midwives. In the context of enabling excellent quality and appropriate care for individual women, the research findings held a strongly characteristic pattern. The findings reflected those of the relationships between independent midwives and supervisors of midwives. A professional relationship was enabling and facilitative on the woman's behalf if the professionals shared a similar ideology of birth and if midwifery practice was accepted as professional rather than semi-professional practice in which midwives exercise clinical judgement and are accountable for their practice. The relationship became increasingly obstructive as ideologies and understanding of midwifery practice diverged. Supervisors of midwives and GPs were experienced as the most obstructive group of professional colleagues by these independent midwives.

Independent midwives views of future of midwifery

These independent midwives were very much ahead of their time and were the forerunners of the organizational changes of midwifery services initially explored in 'The Vision' (Association of Radical Midwives paper published in the 1980s). This particular ideology of pregnancy, birth, midwifery practice and organization of midwifery practice and maternity services, was eventually adopted as government policy in 1993 with the publication of 'Changing Childbirth' (Department of Health, 1993). They represent a 'bridge' between a medicalized maternity service and a woman centred maternity service. These midwives articulated their experience of being a 'signpost' to these changes through sharing their vision of the future of midwifery in the maternity services.

All of the midwives recognized that the then organization of maternity services was stressing for childbearing women and their professional carers alike. They suggested ways forward to create a system where the women are more in control and the professional groups are used appropriately. They were aware of the tensions within the midwifery profession as well as between professional groups. Some were despairing, a few were excited and hopeful, while most sat tensely on the brink of change doing their uttermost to effect a positive change as they saw it.

Two thirds of the midwives saw the way forward as:

- a choice of continuity of carer for women
- community based practice
- organization of midwives into 'teams' or group practices
- women having real choice of place of birth
- midwife practitioners being equivalent and equal to medical practitioners.

Independent midwives: Follow up discussions 1995

It has proved difficult to facilitate discussions with larger groups of independent midwives. Many independent midwives have had to stop their practice during 1994 and 1995 following changes in insurance arrangements for professional practice. The effect was to isolate them as a discrete group, with higher financial risks, in the insurance markets. There was a resultant enormous rise in annual premiums (approximately £5000 per annum), a financial burden, which despite strenuous negotiations was not spread across the total midwifery membership of the Royal College of Midwives. The five year timetable for reorganizing the maternity services (Department of Health, 1993) into a woman centred service has also provided some creative opportunities for a few independent midwives. One practice, The South East London Group Practice, has become a 'provider unit' contracted as an integral part of NHS service provision. They continue to be independent contractors rather than employees. This is a similar arrangement to the family doctor service, they are within the NHS. Since the original research, many of the findings have indeed proved to be 'prophetic' reflecting the position of independent midwifery in the late 1980s as being a forerunner of one of the largest changes in the organization of midwifery services in recent times.

The English National Board for Nursing, Health Visiting and Midwifery (ENB) acknowledged the lack of sufficient knowledge of supervision by many supervisors themselves which resulted in poor role models and a relative invisibility of supervision as a process. They addressed this situation through producing an Open Learning programme, in 1992, to be undertaken by all midwives in England who were nominated as supervisors of midwives. During 1996, the midwifery professional bodies continue this debate regarding the role and realization of supervision as a professional process. The UKCC has strengthened the profile of supervision. The ENB is completing a comprehensive review of its successful open learning programme for preparation of supervisors. The new pack moves forward and addresses the increasing centrality of improving the quality of service provision for women and their families, professional leadership and 'political' negotiation at local level. The Royal College of Midwives published its position statement regarding supervision in midwifery in May 1996. Structurally a major change occurs on April 1st 1996 when the Local Supervisory Authority function transfers to the local Health Commission (the purchasers of health care).

I have collated insights shared during discussion with some midwives who are or had been practising independently. There was agreement that the 'Changing Childbirth' initiative has adopted a similar ideology to that of independent midwifery practice which has been expressed in the phrase 'woman centred service'. This philosophical change is being translated into organizational transition which is required to effect a woman centred service provision. The process has highlighted constraints to midwifery practice which are similar to those experienced previously by independent midwives. The conclusion to be drawn from these constraints is that there must be *control of midwifery professional practice in order to create the conditions in which midwives may be professionally accountable.*

If midwifery is to regain control of professional practice, resources and constraints need to be identified. A central constraint which affects this organizational transition is that the government of the day stated that it had to take place as 'cost neutral'. This meant that all changes have to be funded within existing budgets. Midwifery entered the organizational change with many constraints, before services even began to address developmental costs. These constraints include midwifery 'establishments' (the number of staff which could be employed to provide midwifery services in a district) which had already been eroded during preparation of hospitals for NHS Trust status. These establishments were 'inherited'; they had rarely been planned in any systematic way to reflect the midwifery work that had to be provided. Some effects of this constraint was that midwives workloads have been onerous and impossible to achieve without compromise of quality of service provision and/or individual midwives quality of life. Many midwifery services find it difficult to be able to provide even the basic equipment for all midwives to be able to practice. For example, the sharing of fetal sonicaids, equipment for use when attending a woman birthing at home and even equipment for communication like message pagers or mobile phones. Independent midwives purchased their own equipment and are accountable for the maintenance and replacement. The organization of an institution in these circumstances mitigates against individual accountability and spreads that accountability through several layers i.e. individual practitioners, ward managers, midwifery managers, supervisors of midwives and risk management teams. A cultural change is needed in the NHS to enable midwives to change their place of work. As midwives reorganize into Group Practices or teams often there is no space for them to have an office base. Prior to 'Changing Childbirth', many community midwives did not have an office space of their own in the community and many were crammed into one tiny office in the hospital site. Independent midwives valued being able to have their 'offices' whether they were based in homes or rented accommodation. They valued themselves and had control of their practice base. A further constraint is the financial reward system for midwifery practice. Midwifery being included in the Clinical Grading structure was and remains a controversial arrangement to midwives. A financial system based on nursing structure and practice is not necessarily transferable to midwifery practitioners and their organization of practice. The 'Changing Childbirth' reorganization further stresses this anomaly since the organizational change clarifies that anyone registered and working as a midwife is expected to be accountable as a practitioner. As midwives' job descriptions, employment contracts and work patterns change to facilitate a woman centred maternity service, there is increasing tension in the perpetuation of pay differentials through Clinical Grading structure which does not reflect changed contracts and midwives becoming truly accountable practitioners. The last identified constraint concerns control of practice through establishing guidelines, standards and audit of professional practice. Previously, few individual midwives were involved in this process and therefore had little ownership of their own practice. This organizational model did not encourage a climate of reflective practice or individual accountability. All professionals and user representatives need to be equally involved in this process if a climate of individual accountability and ownership of the maternity services is to be facilitated.

Conclusion

The cost neutral status of the government policy placed the final constraint on the five year developmental plan. Even as the maternity services responsibly identify the gaps to be filled (education and training needs for practitioners to skill or reskill them, relocating service delivery has implications on staffing numbers), they have been placed in a financial impasse. Independent midwives had control of their budget and decision making concerning the services they provided. They were directly accountable for their budget. Midwifery budgets are devolved from the Trust total budget for health service provision. Another layer of accountability and control is in place.

Supervision of midwives is essentially about the quality of the service provided. It is a statutory mechanism which has the potential to enable midwives to have control of their professional practice. During organizational transition, supervision could have two separate but complementary functions to realize this goal. Firstly, it concerns supporting midwives as individual practitioners through 'midwifing the midwives'. Secondly, the supervisory function could be exercised 'politically'. Supervisors have a statutory remit which is beyond that of an employee in an organization. They have a responsibility for monitoring midwifery practice and identifying constraints through audit. For example, they may collate clinical risk management findings, recruitment and retention data and data regarding midwifery education and skilling. Supervision needs to become accountable and visible. Previously it has been rather invisible or limited. Supervisors should then negotiate, and if necessary, lobby appropriate stakeholders (Hospital and Community Trusts, Health Commissions and MSLC's, professional governing bodies and professional organizations) to effect necessary change. This may be seen as 'midwifing midwifery practice'.

The midwifery profession needs to be singularly united and visionary regarding the place of supervisory function in the 21st century. The current arrangements for supervision have the potential to 'midwife' the organizational transition to enable midwives to have control over their professional practice. Midwifery should accept the mantle of reflective practice, peer review and multidisciplinary audit. The norm for professional practice then is the midwife as an autonomous practitioner. Whilst this is being achieved our profession needs to have the foresight to plan an accountable system which has, as its remit, to sustain an excellent quality midwifery service. This system whichever shape it takes must have a high profile and be owned and accepted in the maternity services by all the stakeholders. It is only in this way that such a system may be truly accountable. Eventually supervision in its current form should become redundant and the different functions of supervision could be fulfilled through different routes.

References

Briggs, R. (1989). *Disciplinary Proceedings, Some Lessons from Recent Cases.*

Cartwright, A. (1979). *The Dignity of Labour?* London: Tavistock.

Cronk, M. (1988). 'Midwives must be allowed to exercise clinical judgement' (correspondence) *Nursing Times* 84 (51) 21 December.

Department of Health (1993). *Part 1 Report of the Expert Maternity Group.* London: HMSO.

Fern, A. (1991). *The Vanishing Midwife* unpublished MSc thesis. London: London School of Economics.

Flint, C. (1985). 'Trouble and strife' *Nursing Times* 6 November.

Flint, C. (1987). 'Conflicting allegiances' *Nursing Times* 87 (5) 4 February.

Garcia, J. (1982). 'Women's views of antenatal care' In: Enkin, M., Chalmers, I. (Eds). *Effectiveness and Satisfaction in Antenatal Care.* London: Spastics International Medical Publication. Heinmann Medical Books.

Graham, H., McKee, L. (1979). *The First Months of Motherhood.* Report of a Health Education Council Project concerned with women's' experiences of pregnancy, childbirth and first months of life. Unpublished. York University

Hughes, D. (1985). 'Midwives in trouble: Report on a study day in London' *Association of Radical Midwives Magazine.* Spring

Isherwood, K. (1988). 'Friend or watchdog?' *Nursing Times* 84 (24) 15 June.

Lansdell, M. (1989). 'Friend and counsellor' *Nursing Times* 85 (28) July.

Martin, D.L. (1990). 'The control of reproduction: Law medicine and women. Midwives: Subjects and Agents: A study of social control'. Copy of paper available from 1 Ingleside Grove, Blackheath, London .

Oakley, A. (1979). *Becoming a Mother.* Oxford. Martin Robinson

Reid, M. (1986). 'Non medical aspects in the evaluation of prenatal care for women at low risk'. In: Kaminski, H., Breart, G., Buekers, P. et al. (Eds). *Perinatal Care Delivery Systems. Description and evaluation in European Community Countries.* Oxford: Oxford University Press

Reid, M., McIlwaine, G. (1982). *A Comparison of the Delivery of Antenatal Care between a Hospital and a Peripheral Clinic.* Glasgow: University of Glasgow.

Robinson, S. (1985a). 'Normal maternity care, whose responsibility?' *British Journal of Obstetrics and Gynaecology,* 92: 1-3.

Robinson, S. (1985b). 'Maternity care: a duplication of resources'. *Journal of Royal College General Practitioners,* 35: 346-347

UKCC (1984). *Code of Professional Practice.* London: UKCC.

Warren, C. (1988). 'Scared to be midwives?' *Association of Radical Midwives* No. 38, September.

Weitz, R. (1987). *English Midwives and the Association of Radical Midwives.*

Using the Experience
of Other Professions

CHAPTER FOURTEEN

A Case for Clinical Supervision in Midwifery

Ruth Deery BSc (Hons), RGN, RM, ADM
is a lecturer in the Division of Midwifery and Women's Health, School of Health studies, University of Bradford. She has worked as a midwife for sixteen years and a lecturer for the past three years. She has particular interests in the role of women in society, the concept of empowerment and clinical supervision.

Debi Corby Bsc (Hons), RGN, RMN, Dip N
is a lecturer and course leader in the Division of Nursing Studies, School of Health Studies, University of Bradford. She has worked as a nurse in general and community mental health nursing for over ten years. She has particular interests in women and mental health, the concept of hope and clinical supervision.

Clinical supervision is a much misunderstood and often confusing concept, particularly in the field of midwifery, with many health professionals assuming that the supervisor of midwives provides clinical supervision. In fact, there is a danger that supervisors of midwives may believe they are providing clinical supervision and midwives may believe that they are receiving it, when in reality they are not. Therefore, without clarification of the term and understanding of the concept of clinical supervision, there is a possibility that midwives and the women they care for, will fail to gain the benefits from the experience that is available to them.

One of the main causes of this confusion appears to relate to the use of the term 'supervisor'. This view is reinforced by the United Kingdom Central Council in a recent position document, which states that the term is both misleading and unhelpful (UKCC, 1995). There is no doubt that the confusion is compounded by the abundance of terms with which it is associated. Terms such as: assessor, preceptor, mentor, supervisor, clinical educator/assessor appear to be used interchangeably without consistent understanding. Heagerty (1986) goes some way towards addressing this by referring to this confusion as a 'definition quagmire' and suggests there is a need for standardization of these terms. Some health professionals consider clinical supervision has its roots in midwifery (Butterworth, 1992; Thomas, 1995) with Bishop (1994) actually stating that clinical supervision has been compulsory in midwifery for some 90 years. This further compounds the confusion which exists.

The UKCC (1994) has stated that supervisors of midwives must be registered midwives with experience in clinical midwifery. Those who undertake the role are usually senior midwifery managers within the Health Authority and as such provide supervision of midwives within a formal supervisory structure.

Whilst it can be argued that midwifery does have a long history of compulsory and statutory supervision, which is unique to the United Kingdom, it is clearly evident that this system of supervision is poorly understood by many health professionals who do not recognize the fundamental differences in supervision structures/models and believe that midwives actually engage in clinical supervision. Indeed, Thomas (1995) has pointed out that midwifery supervision has not developed into a model in which midwives become empowered and instead only offers guidance and protection to ensure practice is correct.

The Midwives Act was originally enacted in 1902 to protect the public from unsafe midwifery practice (Bent, 1992). The Act established a public watchdog function, by establishing the statutory role of the supervisor of midwives, which has, in the main, remained unchanged. However, over recent years the role appears to have developed to include counselling, support, friendship and guidance, as well as the established statutory contradictions within the role and relationship, for both supervisors of midwives and midwives. In 1993 the Association of Radical Midwives (ARM) set up a working party to outline and clarify their ideas for the future of midwifery supervision, in the hope that from this a model of supervision would develop which 'is more acceptable to everyone concerned' (ARM, 1995).

For these reasons the authors feel it is important to describe and develop our understanding of the concept of clinical supervision and identify the roles of the clinical supervisor and supervisee within the clinical supervisory relationship. Discussion around the benefits of clinical supervision and clarification of some of the areas of overlap within midwifery (see Table 14.1), which cause continued confusion for many midwives and other health professionals, will also take place.

The role of the clinical supervisor differs from	The role of the supervisee differs from
1a) the role of a **supervisor of midwives** in that the role of the clinical supervisor does not have as its prime focus statutory and 'policing' issues	1b) the role of the **midwife** who is consulting a supervisor of midwives in that they are not requesting external evaluation of a statutory professional issue
2a) the role of a **teacher**, in that the clinical supervisor does not have as its prime focus curriculum content, although some education may take place	2b) the role of the **student**, in that they do not have as their prime focus curriculum issues
3a) the role of the **manager**, in that the clincial supervisor does not have as its prime focus organizational and managerial issues although it must be acknowledged these areas may be discussed	3b) the role of the **midwife** who is being managed in that the prime focus is not organizational but individual issues

Table 14.1: Clarification of role differences (compiled by authors, 1995)

In addition, we offer recommendations and a possible route (see Table 14.2) which may provide a basis for those midwives intending to adopt the concept of clinical supervision within their midwifery practice.

---

1. Explore and clarify your understanding of the concept 'clinical supervision'.

2. Compare and contrast a clinical supervision model with other models of support, including that of the Supervisor of Midwives.

3. Discuss and debate the benefits of clinical supervision with others.

4. Reflect upon your expectations of clinical supervision.

5. Select a clinical supervisor - this may be achieved through 'word of mouth recommendations' or a directory of practising supervisors may be complied and made available to assist this selection process.

6. Arrange an introductory meeting so that roles, responsibilities and expectations can be identified.

7. Negotiate a contract, which will determine the boundaries and barriers to clinical supervision.

8. Negotiate practical arrangements, for example, location, duration, frequency etc.

9. Determine how long your relationship with this clinical supervisor will last.

10. Plan time to evaluate how the clinical supervision process is evolving.

11. Share your experiences of the clinical supervision process with the wider professional group.

12. Reflect upon the impact of clinical supervision within your clinical practice.

Table 14.2: The route to successful and effective clinical supervision (compiled by the authors, 1995)

Clinical supervision

Clinical supervision has been defined by Butterworth (1992) as:

> 'An exchange between practising professionals to enable the development of professional skills' (p.12)

However, we contend, that this definition, although one of the better ones, still fails to provide a 'visual picture' of what clinical supervision encompasses and may add to the confusion by failing to define what is meant by practising professionals. We would like to stress that clinical supervision is not about the mentoring and assessing of students or subordinates, it is broader and should be available to anyone who wishes to develop their personal and/or professional skills. Therefore, to clarify the 'picture' for midwives, we would offer and expand upon Butterworth's (1992) definition by stating that clinical supervision should involve:

> 'time for two people to develop a relationship, in a safe, supportive, relaxed and open environment, with the purpose of using the contracted time to engage in the facilitation of the personal and professional development of the supervisee.' (Compiled by the authors, 1995)

To enhance further this visual picture of clinical supervision, it may be useful to liken it to a therapeutic counselling scenario, where an individual is supported, within a safe relationship by another to 'help them to help themselves' (Rogers, 1983).

However, clinical supervision is not counselling, in that clinical supervision does not have as its prime focus the promotion of healing (Rogers, 1983), although it must be acknowledged that some healing may take place.

Nevertheless, there are some similarities. For example, skills required by counsellors are also required by clinical supervisors. These skills may include: affirming, questioning, challenging, clarifying and focusing. Furthermore, the true spirit of clinical supervision is time for, and with the supervisee in the same way as counselling is client centred.

This contrasts with the supervisor of midwives who although, supporting and caring for the midwife, cannot provide the safe relationship required for clinical supervision as they have a managerial, investigatory and disciplinary role. This could also be referred to as 'the policing role' (Walton, 1995).

Close examination of the Midwives Rules (UKCC, 1993, rule 44, p.22) shows that the supervisor of midwives is appointed to be 'over' the midwife rather than 'with' the midwife. Therefore, the safe relationship required for clinical supervision is threatened by the superior and hierarchical nature of the supervisor of midwives role.

Furthermore, Rogers (1983) suggests that for relationships to be therapeutic - they should be free from external evaluation. That is, the considerations and judgements of others should not influence the nature and development of the relationship. Curtis (1992) states that one of the roles of the supervisor of midwives, within their formal supervisory structure, is to 'bring the distant professional hierarchy to bear upon the daily practice of clinical midwifery'. Mayes (1993) states that the role of the supervisor of midwives includes 'the exercising of professional judgement to reach conclusions about safe practice'. Therefore, this 'bearing upon' and 'exercising' further restricts the ability of the supervisor of midwives to provide the safe relationship as they are forced to make external evaluations.

The individual who takes on the role of 'supervisor of midwives' may be an experienced midwife, guide, counsellor and friend and although it is recognized that this role is a crucial and necessary one, we believe it is fraught with difficulties that contradict the true spirit and core conditions of clinical sup .vision. Indeed, the question must be asked, who supports the supervisor of midwives when she is expected to carry out this multi-faceted role? As the role has developed there appears to have been no consideration given to the support the supervisor of midwives may desire. Although the local supervising authorities (LSAs) are available (Mayes, 1993), the question arises as to whether the type of support accessible is not only what the supervisor of midwives requires, but also whether it is relevant to clinical supervision. Therefore we believe that supervisors of midwives are not in the best position to act as clinical supervisors as it places unfair and unforeseen demands and dilemmas upon them.

The true spirit of clinical supervision involves the establishing of a safe forum through the development of a therapeutic relationship. By their very nature these relationships are based upon conditions of trust, warmth, openness and honesty or care, acceptance, regard and empathy (Rogers, 1983). These conditions derive from the conviction that the other is trustworthy, dependable, accepting, sensitive and consistent.

The conditions, referred to above, do not 'just happen' but require certain skills, attitudes and beliefs on the part of both individuals. It may be assumed that professionals, who work within nursing and midwifery, by the very fact that they have been trained and educated to work with others, possess these skills. However, we agree with Taylor (1994) who in the continuing debate on clinical supervision suggests that the required skills are not part of the present knowledge base of nurses and midwives and need to be developed. Therefore, we strongly recommend that an additional period of training or education should be undertaken. This should be available to both clinical supervisors and supervisees to further develop their understanding and expectations of the skills required for clinical supervision.

Furthermore, we believe clinical supervision should be formal in nature with regard to allocated time. That is, with both parties aware of the practical arrangements for the relationship. The practical details of how often, where and how long are crucially important as clinical supervision should not be on an 'ad hoc' basis. This endangers the therapeutic nature of the relationship and fails to acknowledge the importance of the time and privacy necessary for the creation of a safe environment. For example, an agreement may be reached to meet fortnightly, for one hour, at a neutral location.

In addition, this agreement should also address the 'ending' of the relationship. It is important that neither the clinical supervisor nor the supervisee feel obligated to maintain a relationship that may have lost its value and has taken the form of 'sitting with Nellie' as described by Burnard (1990). By addressing the 'ending' at the beginning of the relationship, both parties can openly discuss the dangers of dependency and the opportunities of working with others without feeling a sense of rejection.

Therefore, it is crucial that both parties identify their beliefs and negotiate the structure and form their relationship may take. As well as including the practical details, key issues of confidentiality, responsibility, autonomy and risk taking should also be addressed.

Agreed arrangements should be made early within the relationship as they are crucial in establishing the boundaries and barriers within the therapeutic relationship which may develop as a result. We advocate that each of these issues is negotiated and formally contracted as failure to do so may threaten the safety of the midwives concerned and their professional standing. For example, if a supervisee shares a professional concern with her supervisor which is in breach of local protocols, it then needs to be established whose responsibility it is to take that matter further? If the clinical supervisor independently takes this matter further, the confidence and trust of the supervisee may be lost. These matters need to be acknowledged as potential areas for concern, and strategies negotiated and in place to deal with them. By doing this there would be an acknowledgement of professional boundaries and consequences of failing to honour these boundaries for both the clinical supervisor and supervisee. It is important to note that there are some boundaries which cannot be crossed, for example illegal and/or unethical practice, and both parties need to acknowledge their responsibilities with regard to this. These negotiated and agreed strategies would help to create a facilitative climate where each could clarify agendas and the potential constraints to the core conditions (for example, confidentiality) that their professional responsibilities place upon them.

Such negotiations may help to clarify the position of the supervisor of midwives – who may suggest that the supervisee forms an additional relationship with a clinical supervisor as well as maintaining the relationship with herself. This will ensure that statutory requirements are complied with. A recent research study by Fowler (1995), which explored nurses' perceptions of the elements of good clinical supervision, demonstrated that students believe that a clinical supervisor should be 'knowledgeable in the areas in which the student wishes to develop expertise'. However, it must be noted that a midwife may elect to receive clinical supervision from a supervisor who is not a midwife. Whilst this idea of crossing professional boundaries may be met by initial anxiety, it must be noted, that to some midwives, it may be more important that the clinical supervisor possesses the necessary therapeutic and facilitation skills for effective clinical supervision. Once boundaries and barriers to clinical supervision, such as this, are addressed, roles and responsibilities will be identified, and the therapeutic relationship can begin to be established.

The role of the clinical supervisor

The role of the clinical supervisor is to facilitate personal and professional growth and development in the supervisee. The clinical supervisor provides a forum, which encourages free expression of any concerns, ambitions, strengths and deficiencies of the supervisee, and responds to them in an accepting, open and supportive manner.

The clinical supervisor may be best placed to constructively challenge supervisees to reflect on their actions (Schon, 1983) in both the relationship of clinical supervision and relationships outside of the clinical supervision process. The clinical supervisor therefore has a role in centring the relationship on 'the here and now' (Hawkins and Shohet, 1989). This will provide the opportunity for the supervisees to engage in reflective practice, thereby gaining insight into how they currently, and may in the future, interact with others. This may involve the clinical supervisor acting as a resource for the supervisee by providing information based upon their observations of the supervisee within the relationship and through drawing upon their own clinical experiences and knowledge. The clinical supervisor also has a responsibility to reflect upon their own personal and professional growth. This reflection should include consideration and evaluation of their experience as a clinical supervisor and this may take place within their own clinical supervision network/relationship.

The role of the supervisee

Kirkham (1994) states that there are two reasons why midwives need clinical supervision. The first is to acknowledge their need to 'practice from a secure basis in the face of vulnerability, change and uncertainty'. The second is the need for guidance, support and inspiration of their practice.

Therefore, the role of the supervisee in clinical supervision is to use the time and skills of the clinical supervisor to aid their own personal and professional growth and development. This may mean that the supervisee needs to acknowledge their own vulnerabilities, the changes and uncertainties with which they are faced and the impact this may have upon their current midwifery practice. They also have a responsibility to be prepared to identify and prioritise these issues for discussion.

The supervisee must also be prepared to engage in reflection and exploration. Through reflection the supervisee will be in a position to identify how they can build upon their strengths and request guidance and inspiration for areas of practice they wish to develop further.

Supervisors also have a responsibility to consider their experience of participating in a clinical supervisory relationship, as this will provide them with a forum to examine how they relate and react to others, receive feedback and provide a safe environment where they can rehearse and evaluate their interpersonal skills.

The benefits of clinical supervision

Clinical supervision is concerned with people and not tasks (Lawton, 1987) and therefore could be viewed as effective in empowering both midwives and women in their care. The notion of empowerment is particularly pertinent in the ideas expressed in 'The Named Midwife' (Department of Health, 1992a) and the Government Response (Department of Health, 1992b) to the 'Second Report, Maternity Services' (House of Commons Health Committee, 1992).

Furthermore:

1. It helps individuals to become aware of their strengths, prejudices and areas for future development.
2. It may also provide a place to regain some of the energy that is lost when individuals use themselves as a resource – which occurs by the very nature of working with people therapeutically (Lawton, 1987).
3. It has a protective function which can provide a professional support system against stress and burnout (Faugier, 1992).
4. It may serve as a preventative measure against the isolation and solitude experienced by many midwives, particularly those in a community setting (Thomas, 1995).
5. The relationship established may serve as a point of reference for the development of relationships with others, with the clinical supervisor acting as a role model, and both parties exploring issues of relationship development (Oxley, 1995).
6. It provides a forum where learning takes place, with the opportunity to reflect upon clinical practice, and the integration of theoretical knowledge and research into future clinical practice.

Conclusion

As a consequence of the benefits of clinical supervision there may be advantages for all people with whom midwives are associated. This may include: mothers, babies, their families, fellow professionals, students and the wider professional group. Through these benefits there may be increased opportunities to develop and enhance midwifery care through innovative and reflective practice.

Clinical supervision is an area of crucial importance to the midwifery profession. When offered and used effectively it can provide midwives with the opportunity not only to improve and extend their clinical expertise but it may provide them with a framework to increase understanding of what it means to them personally, to be an empowered and empowering midwife in the 1990s.

This chapter has addressed issues relating to what the authors believe will build upon and enhance clinical supervision as a concept within today's midwifery arena. Our intention has been to offer an effective and practical model, which we believe will enhance safe and accountable midwifery practice where new patterns in the way midwifery care is organized have placed additional responsibilities and stresses upon midwives.

It is hoped the model offered here will be considered, discussed and piloted by midwives meeting the current challenge to adopt appropriate and workable models of clinical supervision. The authors would welcome comments, feedback and research-based evidence to continue to add the body of knowledge on clinical supervision in the 1990s.

Recommendations

1. All midwives should explore the concept of clinical supervision and decide for themselves if and how clinical supervision may enhance their personal and professional development. Rodgers (1989) has suggested that unless a concept is considered significant, it will not be used often and will stifle the development of productive innovations.

2. Clinical supervision should be planned, evaluated and researched by the midwives who engage in it and by other interested parties.

3. Adequate funding and resources should be made available to allow for the implementation and evaluation of clinical supervision in midwifery practice.

4. Training and education needs of midwives involved in offering and receiving clinical supervision should be further identified and included in midwifery training and education programmes.

5. The professional and personal benefits of clinical supervision should be measured in terms of the effect of individual and organizational changes.

6. Further discussion is necessary to review the continuing trend for the hierarchical and compulsory nature of supervision within current midwifery practice.

7. Changing the role of the supervisor of midwives may be inevitable in the light of our evolving model of clinical supervision in midwifery. We recommend therefore, the greatest change should be seen in allowing the supervisor of midwives to focus upon the statutory aspects of their role and clinical supervisors to focus upon the safe, therapeutic relationship with midwife.

8. A prerequisite for establishing a clinical supervision relationship should be the negotiation of a contract to identify issues of responsibility, accountability, confidentiality in order that the dilemmas of a hierarchical and potentially judgmental relationship are avoided. This would ensure that the relationship taking place is of a therapeutic nature.

9. To position clinical supervision high on the midwifery professions agenda there is a need for, not only personal evaluations, but also the inclusion of rigorous research-based evidence of its effectiveness.

References

Association of Radical Midwives (1994). 'Future midwifery supervision'. *Midwifery Matters,* Spring, 60, pp.25-28.

Association of Radical Midwives (1995). 'Super-Vision'. *Midwifery Matters,* 65, Summer, pp.13-14.

Bent, E.A. (1992). *The Statutory Basis to the Role of Supervisor.* Module 1, Preparation of Supervisors of Midwives. London: ENB.

Bishop, V. (1994). 'Clinical supervision for an accountable profession'. *Nursing Times,* 28 September, 90, 39, pp.35-37.

Burnard, P. (1990). 'The student experience: adult learning and mentorship revisited'. *Nurse Education Today,* 10, pp.349–54.

Butterworth, T. (1992). 'Clinical supervision as an emerging idea in nursing'. In: Butterworth, T., Faugier, J. (Eds). *Clinical Supervision and Mentorship in Nursing.* London: Chapman and Hall.

Curtis, P. (1992). 'Supervision in clinical midwifery practice'. In: Butterworth, T., Faugier, J. (Eds). *Clinical Supervision and Mentorship in Nursing.* London: Chapman and Hall.

Department of Health (1992a). *The Named Midwife.* London: HMSO.

Department of Health (1992b). *Maternity Services, Government Response to the Second Paper from the Health Committee Session 1991–92.* London: HMSO.

Fowler, J. (1995). 'Nurses' perceptions of the elements of good supervision'. *Nursing Times*, 91, 22, p.37.

Heagerty, B. (1986). 'A second look at mentors: do you really need one to succeed in nursing?' *Nursing Outlook*, 34, 1, January/February, pp.16-19, 24.

Hawkins, P. (1982). 'Mapping it out'. *Community Care*, 22 July, pp.17-19.

Hawkins, P., Shohet, R. (1989). *Supervision in the Helping Professions.* Milton Keynes: Open University Press.

HMSO (1992). *Second Report, Maternity Service.* House of Commons Health Committee, Chaired by N. Winterton. London: HMSO.

Isherwood, K. (1988). 'Friend or watchdog?' *Nursing Times*, 84, 24, p.65.

Kirkham, M. (1994). 'Super-Vision, a contribution to the debate'. *Midwifery Matters*, 60, Spring, p.27.

Lawton, D. (1987). *Supervision – A System of Personal Supervision for Student Nurses, Students and Supervisors Handbook.* Unpublished. Leeds: Highroyds Hospital.

Mayes, G. (1993). 'Quality through supervision'. *British Journal of Midwifery*, 1, 3, pp.138-41.

Oxley, P. (1995). 'Clinical supervision in community psychiatric nursing'. *Mental Health Nursing*, 15, 6, pp.29-32.

Rodgers, B.L. (1989). 'Concepts, analysis and the development of nursing knowledge: the evolutionary cycle'. *Journal of Advanced Nursing*, Vol. 14, pp.330-35.

Rogers, C. (1983). *Freedom to Learn for the 80s.* New York: Merrill.

Schon, D.A. (1983). *The Reflective Practitioner.* New York: Basic Books.

Taylor, M. (1994). 'Continuing the debate on supervision, the supervision of midwives'. *Midwifery Matters,* 60, Spring, p.28.

Thomas, S. (1995). 'Clinical supervision'. *Journal of Community Nursing*, October, pp.12-18.

UKCC (1993). *Midwives Rules.* London: UKCC.

UKCC (1994). *A Midwife's Code of Practice.* London: UKCC.

UKCC (1995). 'Clinical supervision for Nursing and Health Visiting'. *Registrar's Letter* 4/95, 24 January. London: UKCC.

Walton, I. (1995). 'Conflicts in supervision of midwives'. In: Association of Radical Midwives (Eds). *Super-Vision, Consensus Conference Proceedings.* Hale: Books for Midwives Press, pp.31-38.

CHAPTER FIFTEEN

An Ex-Midwife's Reflections on Supervision from a Psychotherapeutic Viewpoint

Meg Taylor Bsc, MSc, RM, Dip Couns
is a psychodynamic counsellor and therapist and was accredited by the British Association for Counselling in 1994. She trained as a direct entry midwife and worked for seven years in both hospital and community, after which time she gained a diploma in Counselling and Interpersonal Skills at the Institute of Education. Her particular interest is in the emotional aspects of childbirth and their impact on midwifery training and practice.

In this chapter I aim to raise a number of questions which I hope will be relevant to midwives in their efforts to develop a system of supervision which will suit their profession. I do not aim to provide any answers; this would not be appropriate from someone who is now outside the profession. Also I do not have any answers: what follows is intended to be speculative.

I now work as a counsellor and a psychotherapist. There is no consensus in counselling or psychotherapy about what distinguishes the two. My working definition is that counselling is short term and focused and psychotherapy is open ended and therefore does not need to be so structured. In Britain at the moment there are two main regulatory bodies, the British Association for Counselling (BAC) and the United Kingdom Council for Psychotherapy (UKCP), but members of BAC include those who consider themselves psychotherapists and some practitioners hold joint membership.

I believe the words 'counselling' and 'psychotherapy' express a clear hierarchical relationship. Ben Lawrence of the UKCP stated (personal communication, 1995) 'psychotherapy is based at postgraduate level and courses last a minimum of three years'.

Counselling is open to those without degree level qualifications. The counselling course I did only required students to be engaged in work, voluntary or paid, which involved the use of counselling skills. I mention this because I think these differences in educational requirement and the consequent differences in status mirror the relationship between midwifery and obstetrics.

Counselling and psychotherapy are however completely unregulated professions. Membership of BAC or UKCP is entirely voluntary, they are not equivalent to the UKCC or GMC. The BAC provides a code of ethics and practice to which all practising members must adhere and this includes a clear commitment to supervision. The amount of supervision will depend on the size of the caseload, but supervision is an ongoing undertaking, it does not end with qualification. The UKCP covers a much more multifarious membership. Its member organizations range from psychoanalytic psychotherapists to hypnotherapists and those who practice body or art therapy. It does not specify that therapists must be in supervision, although individual member organizations may require their own members to continue in supervision. This will depend on their underlying philosophy and orientation. It is my distinct impression that psychoanalytic psychotherapists frequently view supervision as a part of training, although they may return to supervision after qualification at times when particular problems in practice are isolated. My own supervisor told me that she went through a period after qualifying when she had no supervision and found the experience liberating: she used it as an opportunity to work out her own personal style of practice.

There are two models here. One where supervision is seen as intrinsic to practice, and another where it is seen primarily as an aspect of training. To return to the analogy with midwifery and obstetrics, it seems to me that midwives are far more supervised, both formally through the statutory supervisory process and informally through line management and by policies and procedures, than obstetricians who allow themselves wider clinical judgement. Some years ago, a London teaching hospital required its student midwives to witness a number of births before they could deliver their first baby, while the medical students had no such requirement. The questionable reasoning seemed to be that the higher academic level of medicine implied a better grasp of theory and therefore less need for practice. Within the unstated hierarchy of counselling and psychotherapy, psychoanalytic psychotherapists come highest and I wonder if a similar reasoning applies. In other words, is there an unspoken assumption that the higher the theoretical educational and professional status, the less need for supervision?

It is evident from Heagerty's chapter in this book that supervision developed to control and limit the practice of lay midwives who were seen as threatening for a number of reasons. They threatened the political aim of the Victorian ladies whose ideas of achieving change were limited to doing so through using men's power, by allying midwifery to medicine as an auxiliary and inferior profession. They were also threatening precisely because they were poor and often illiterate. People in oppressed groups bear, in addition to their physical oppression, the extra burden of being on the receiving end of projection. In Victorian society those qualities which the middle classes preferred not to acknowledge came to be seen as the special province of the poor. The qualities most usually denied and projected are sexual potency and aggression. The poor are then disproportionately feared - and envied - because of their dangerous sexuality and potential for violence.

This mechanism is as evident today as in the last century, when certain groups, especially the 'underclass' and ethnic minorities are seen to carry characteristics which the in group denies it possesses. Members of these groups may come to accept and internalize the projections put on to them. Projection will also flow the other way; for example the oppressed group may come to internalize powerlessness and see the oppressing group as all-powerful.

I don't know to what extent a similar motive underlies the history of supervision in counselling and psychotherapy. My supervisor joked that it developed initially because Freud could not relinquish control over his followers' work. Is there another assumption, probably more pertinent here for midwifery than counselling and psychotherapy, that supervision exists to control, and an implication that if something needs to be controlled it is in some way dangerous? I shall return to these questions.

The debate about the development of midwifery supervision at the moment is taking place in a context where structures of clinical supervision are being developed for nurses and health visitors. Whenever this was raised at the UKCC's briefing meetings, which I attended on behalf of the Association of Radical Midwives (ARM), I was always a little bewildered that midwives' supervision was held up as a model. My bewilderment arose because it seems evident to me that whatever the present statutory arrangement offers midwives, it is not clinical supervision. But I was also bewildered because I was aware of considerable dissatisfaction with midwifery supervision. Some people experienced it as punitive; they only became aware of their supervisors as anything other than the recipient of their intention to practise forms when they were deemed to have done something wrong. Independent midwives in particular according to Demilew (1995), experienced supervision in a 'controlling, negative and obstructive way'. It seemed to me that often midwives were being penalized for practising in a way that put their loyalty to their client and their own clinical judgement above that of formalized general policies; in other words if they practised in a similar manner to that of obstetricians by exercising clinical autonomy.

The concept of clinical autonomy came to seem very important as I thought about supervision and 'Changing Childbirth' (Department of Health, 1993). According to Edwards (1993), this report requires services to be woman centred and accessible to all and tailored to individual needs. Women should 'be able to make an initial booking with GP or midwife; be encouraged to plan their care with the appropriate professionals; be encouraged to think about the birth itself; be enabled to change their booking or plans for birth at any stage during pregnancy; have the right to choose different forms of care; be respected by professionals'. How can midwives deliver this without a repertoire of flexible responses to different women's needs and wishes in different situations? The delivery of this level of care seems clearly incompatible to me with any kind of blanket system of policies and procedures. In other words, midwives must be educated to a level where they can exercise a quality of clinical autonomy analogous to that of obstetricians, although the area within which they make decisions with their clients about care will obviously be entirely different from the area of expertise of obstetricians. They must also have the ongoing trust and support of their colleagues, both midwifery and medical, to do this.

I believe the development of this level of clinical autonomy is problematic within the present professional structure of midwifery, that existing managerial hierarchies and supervisory structures are counterproductive, for reasons which I will amplify.

In addition supervisors of midwives are asked both to police and support their supervisees, often within a context where the roles of supervisor and manager are combined. This seems inevitably to evoke confusion. The BAC Code of Practice states that when the supervisor and manager are the same person, the counsellor must have access to outside consultative support which will be both independent and confidential.

The political context of the recent structural changes in the NHS must also be considered. How can supervisors or managers provide adequate support to midwives if they themselves feel inadequately supported? Many managers in the present political climate of the NHS are in a very difficult position, being required to implement changes with which they may not agree for financial rather than clinical reasons.

Before I attended the ARM consensus conference (ARM, 1995) on supervision in April 1995, I was in two minds about supervision, but both of those minds were quite clear. I thought either that midwives should have no supervision at all, because it is incompatible with true clinical autonomy. Or I thought that midwives should have the kind of supervision I have as a counsellor, supervision which is clinical and supportive and entirely independent of any policing structure. I thought that it would be simple to separate out the policing and support aspects of supervision and that the public would be adequately protected against bad practice by the existence of the UKCC, midwives' line management structures and by clients' being given written copies of their rights, of standards expected and of the complaints procedure.

But I was anxious, as I stated at the conference (Taylor, 1995), whether the midwifery ethos was such that supportive supervisory structures could be developed. My anxiety focused on two areas: a culture within midwifery which can be hierarchical, competitive and punitive, both towards midwives and clients - mothers and babies -and a real lack of resources. With regard to the latter it is a basic tenet of counselling that I cannot be expected to give to my client if I don't feel I have enough resources for myself. Counsellors are expected to make sure they have enough resources to function. This requires a kind of self-centredness which is not egotism but which ultimately serves the interests of the client.

Yet I am not only referring to the kind of psychological resources which counselling supervision exists to provide, but real financial scarcity. I am aware that midwives are being asked to take on the increased personal responsibility and autonomy that 'Changing Childbirth' (Department of Health, 1993) requires without any commensurate change in salary or status. When the clinical grading structures first came out it seemed obvious to me that any midwife working as a 'practitioner in her own right', as I was taught as a student we all should be, must be a G grade. But the hierarchical mentality and limited resources ensured that only senior sisters and community midwives were given G grades. The development of integrated teams of midwives, however beneficial this may be for the client, implies that working in the community, which requires a capacity for independent judgement which only experience can provide and which was previously recognized by a G grade, is now carried out by E and F grades. Instead of recognizing that all midwives need to operate on a higher level to deliver the individualized care that 'Changing Childbirth' requires, it seems that clinical autonomy has itself become downgraded. From my perspective midwives have every right to be cynical and embittered. Scarce resources breed competition and envy, and while I believe we all experience this to some extent, they cannot be the basis for generous and compassionate care, either towards clients or supervisees.

There is debate within psychoanalytic circles about the extent to which envy is innate or acquired. Klein (1975) believed it to be innate while others such as Milner (1987) believe it to be a product of a deficiency in the relationship of a baby and its primary carers. There is no doubt in my mind that envy and competition for resources, both physical and psychological, are fostered in certain organizational structures. Hatton (1994) states 'Difficulties in collaboration arise not so much from the desire to be an ideal carer or a more potent worker but from a sense of being an inevitable loser in a competitive struggle. In the current climate of market values and shrinking budgets, the success of one part of the organization can be felt to be at the expense of another. The survival anxiety of the less successful section stimulates an envious desire to spoil the others success'. Market forces and shrinking budgets describe well the physical scarcity of resources in the NHS at the moment.

In addition a hierarchical structure, with its emphasis on above and below, can induce a sense of psychological scarcity. And midwives work within a culture where self centredness is derided and an impossible ideal of perfection and invulnerability prevails. Hawkins and Shohet (1989) state 'as part of our training we are taught to pay attention to client needs and it is often difficult to focus on our own needs. It is even considered selfish or self indulgent'. Yet Hawkins and Shohet go on to argue persuasively that supervision is worthwhile. They culminate in a quotation from Tonnesmann: 'The human encounter in the helping profession is inherently stressful. The stress aroused can be accommodated and used for the understanding of our patients and clients. But our emotional responsiveness will wither if the human encounter cannot be contained within the institutions in which we work. Defensive manoeuvres will then become operative and these will prevent healing, even if cure can be maintained by scientific methods, technical skills and organizational competence. By contrast, if we can maintain contact with the emotional reality of our clients and ourselves then the human encounter can facilitate not only a hearing experience, but also an enriching experience for them and us'.

When I came to consider this chapter I thought about the kind of support I had experienced as a practising midwife. After I qualified in 1980 I stayed on at my training hospital for six months and felt unobtrusively but consistently supported by my colleagues, especially on the labour ward. It seemed they allowed me to practise as I thought best, and when I made mistakes they were on my side. This support was totally unstructured and certainly was not supervision. I contrasted this memory of subtle support with my experiences of group supervision as a trainee on both a psychotherapy and a counselling course. Although my first supervisor was very experienced and skilled and I felt her to be caring and that her confrontations were compassionate, I was very reluctant to reveal myself through my work. My mistrust was based on an expectation that I and my work would be attacked. This was partly irrational and a product of my past experience and personality. But it was also quite sensible: people in groups do attack each other. In a later group we never came adequately to perform the task of examining our work because the dynamics of envy and competitiveness in the group prevented anyone from feeling safe enough to expose their work. These negative experiences are personal to me, but also reflect feelings which are common in group supervision and which can paralyse and subvert the process. A supervisor needs to be skilled and confident enough to expose the dynamics and deal with them.

I contrasted this feeling of inadequacy in counselling and psychotherapy supervision groups with the unobtrusive sense of support I had felt from my midwifery colleagues after qualifying and I was confused. I continue to believe that counselling and psychotherapy have a much kinder ethos and less authoritarian structure than midwifery, yet my experience of midwives was of care and support and of my fellow trainees in psychotherapy and counselling as potentially attacking. I drew two conclusions.

Firstly, I had to learn to use the process of formal supervision and this learning required me to change as a person, to become more trusting and less competitive and envious myself. Paradoxically surviving in groups where these issues came uncomfortably out into the open was one of the factors that helped me to change.

Secondly, the nature of hierarchical structures encourages a split between attack and support. I stated earlier that my colleagues felt to be on my side. At that time there was a culture of conflicting interests: qualified staff versus students; doctors versus midwives; professionals versus clients. By qualifying I became part of a beleaguered group which could support each other because we defined ourselves in opposition to *them*: students or doctors or clients. I experienced benign support while those in the out-groups experienced attack.

What I am saying here is quite complex: that the hierarchy protects against uncomfortable feelings such as anxiety or envy by encouraging those feelings to be split off and projected out onto other layers of the hierarchy. The counselling and psychotherapy groups, on the other hand, brought these uncomfortable feelings home and by doing so we were forced to confront them and learn that they were survivable.

Menzies-Lyth (1988) in her seminal study of nurses found that nurses experience intense anxiety: their own, their patients' and their patients' relatives'. In order to cope with these levels of anxiety they develop certain psychological defence mechanisms which include denial, splitting and projection and they also work within institutions which are structured in such a way as to encourage these psychological processes. These institutional structures include hierarchy and make possible the specific psychological devices nurses use, which include in Menzies-Lyth's own words: 'Splitting up the nurse/patient relationship..., denial of feelings..., the attempt to eliminate decision making by ritual task performance..., reducing the weight of responsibility by check and counter-checks..., delegation to superiors..., avoidance of change'.

It may be argued that Menzies-Lyth's study is out of date, and it is true that by developing the concepts of total patient care and primary nursing, the nursing profession attempted to redress the shortcomings in care which result from these psychological defences. But I note now, under pressure of financial restraint, the concept of 'skill-mix' has been used in effect to sabotage these concepts. It is not deemed cost-effective for a qualified nurse to give a bedpan.

It may also be argued that nurses are not midwives, and I totally agree with this. However, I was impressed at the consensus conference (ARM, 1995) by the reluctance of many of the delegates to give up the policing aspect of supervision and their reluctance was due to their concern about 'dangerous practitioners'. I think this is a very real concern, but I also think that the incidence of real dangerous practitioners is minuscule, and that this concern reflects something else: real dangers in all midwives' practice; dangers which to some extent differentiate midwifery from nursing. Briefly put, these dangers are death, sex, madness and love.

Nurses of course deal with the threat and actuality of death, but death in midwifery is comparatively rare and I believe, therefore, more taboo. Gecko (1995) referring to an international conference of midwives writes: 'the workshop on overcoming fear in childbirth made me think about issues of control and midwife distress and my worst fears about avoidable death of a baby or a woman. Also recognizing and trying to accept that unavoidable death happens in relationship to pregnancy and childbirth. Naming my fears and being able to talk about them in a loving supportive environment was a process I had not experienced before with other midwives but I feel it needs to be an essential and current part of midwifery practice'.

Childbirth is also inextricable from sexuality: it is undeniably how babies are conceived and I maintain that the experience of pregnancy, labour and breastfeeding are also sexual events. Sexuality is a delicate and intimate and profoundly anxiety-provoking area. Addressing it means to take on other taboos (Southern, 1994).

I also believe midwives confront madness because they are in a constant state either of empathy with or a struggle not to empathise with the peculiar frame of mind childbearing woman experience which Winnicott (1975) called primary material preoccupation. This is a state of absorption with the developing fetus and new baby which is so intense that in other circumstances Winnicott said it would be described as mental illness. This absorption requires a blurring of the mother's sense of self and blurring of the boundaries of the self can be particularly threatening: in other contexts it is called psychosis.

The relationship between mother and baby is arguably the most powerful relationship human beings experience. This intense love can evoke powerful feelings in others: envy of the baby, the care it receives, envy of the mother, the special quality of new motherhood, her possession of the baby, her creativity. Most midwives are women. Those who are already mothers will find their own experiences touched upon, comfortably or not. Those who are not mothers are confronted with this fact, and while some midwives may happily have chosen childlessness others may have a history of infertility, miscarriage or loss of a baby.

I do not believe midwives can encounter the creativity of childbirth without being in some way touched. Lomas (1987) writes: 'I have suggested that one factor in the gruesome charade of the traditional labour ward at its worst is man's envy of woman's ability to be a mother. However, in trying to account for a concealed hostility to maternity one could think in terms of the conflict between men and women, the individual and society, family and the state or the physical and the spiritual. But the conflict that has, I believe, the deepest significance, is that between creativity and sterility'.

Midwives therefore have good reasons to have developed psychological and institutional defences against these dangers. But if they are to implement 'Changing Childbirth' (Department of Health, 1993) they cannot use these defences. Continuity of carer requires a relationship with the client and is incompatible with task allocation. A higher rate of home births means that midwives must learn to feel comfortable practising outside the institution. Individualized care requires flexibility and clinical autonomy and neither midwives nor their managers and supervisors can rely on the inflexibility of written, generalized procedures.

It was in the light of this necessary dismantling of the psychological and institutional defences that I thought good quality supportive and clinical supervision might be crucial.

However, I still felt a nagging discomfort about the parallel between statutory supervision of midwives and its history of control and BAC's insistence on mandatory supervision for counsellors. Is there somewhere an assumption that neither midwives or counsellors are mature or well educated enough to recognize areas of concern in their practice and seek help when necessary? Professions which have true autonomy of practice, the law and medicine, do not seem to require supervision. But these are male dominated professions whose structures might be described as masculine. Menzies-Lyth's denial of feelings is endemic in them. Should they be models for midwives? Maybe the BAC's insistence on supervision does not reflect a mistrust of the counsellor's abilities, but a rejection of the concept of independence and a recognition that we are all interdependent; instead of the lone 'masculine' practitioner we have a pattern of 'feminine' networking. I concluded that perhaps supportive and clinical supervision should be mandatory for midwives as a recognition of their worth and of the fact that 'Changing Childbirth' (Department of Health, 1993) is placing new responsibilities on them. However, to reflect the flexibility of practice that midwives need to adopt, I concluded that styles of supervision should vary. It could be group or individual, with peers or those more advanced in practice, formal or informal. It may include the model used by psychoanalytic psychotherapists that while supervision is necessary for training it may not be necessary after qualification, unless the practitioner is encountering problems. It should certainly reflect the fact that different midwives have different needs from other midwives and that their own needs will change and develop over time.

I put this conclusion to a trusted friend, not a midwife but a nurse, and his immediate response was: help, what about those who don't seek supervision? I am stuck again by this mistrust of midwives. Are there so many practitioners who are dangerous at worst or time-servers at best? And if not, why do people believe there are? This led me to a hard conclusion. The BAC trusts counsellors to seek appropriate supervision and I see no sign among colleagues and friends that this trust is betrayed. Yet the delegates at the consensus conference and the friend I consulted do not trust midwives. I believe that this lack of trust reflects the punitive and persecutory nature of the midwifery hierarchy and its ethos. When aggression is projected outwards on to others there is an unconscious fear that it will return, aimed at oneself.

I also feel that this mistrust is an expression of a contempt which midwives have for themselves and for others and which is an internalization of their inferior position with regard to obstetrics.

In the relationship of midwifery and obstetrics there are many projections in both directions. A recent TV series, Cardiac Arrest, brought home to me with a sense of shock how much the doctors envied the nurses. In this country it is the midwives who deliver the babies, who participate in and facilitate the power and catharsis of normal childbirth. Obstetricians intervene when things go wrong and may thus be ascribed a great potency, but they miss out on the opportunity to build up a continuous relationship and be 'with woman' and both midwives and obstetricians may envy each other for these reasons. Ironically by using the defences Menzies-Lyth described midwives have also, to some extent, missed out on this opportunity. James (1990) describes how she perceives midwives deliberately diluting their physical support of women in labour because they find the emotional heat too great. This defensive pattern which reduces the amount and quality of physical contact between midwife and woman may also be seen as an internalization of obstetric working practices.

I return to the contrast between the counselling and midwifery ethos. Counsellors are unregulated, and yes there are episodes of exploitation and abuse. But on the whole my experience is of a body of conscientious and client-centred practitioners. I may have given an impression earlier of counselling and psychotherapy supervision as a forum for envious attack, but after I had learnt to trust myself, my supervisor and the process I came to derive immense value from it. Sometimes we go through sticky moments, but on the whole I leave a session feeling nourished, enthused and filled with respect for the courage of my clients. It is part of our task, both in counselling and in supervision, to encourage feelings to be aired, confronted and survived. This may seem frightening, and it is, but it is also ultimately strengthening. Counselling supervision provides a supportive structure where I developed the equivalent of clinical autonomy. Could an analogous system midwife midwives through the transition from a hierarchy which encourages delegation upwards to a more egalitarian network structure which will both foster and reflect clinical autonomy?

It is possible that counsellors are, on the whole, conscientious and client centred because they do not work within regulated structures and must therefore accept entirely the responsibility for their own standards of practice. I do believe the vast majority of midwives are conscientious, but I am not sure that they are yet truly client centred. Nor do I believe they can be until their support structures foster the kind of self-centredness described above. The structure of the support system and the underlying ethos have a mutually reinforcing relationship. Hierarchy both produces and is a product of an emotion suppressing ethos. But I do not believe clinical autonomy can flourish unsupported. Lawyers and doctors are secure in their academic underpinnings and their sense of status. This however, can mean a gulf between practitioner and client, a suppression of empathy and a defensive arrogance. Midwives must develop supportive structures which allow both clinical autonomy and empathy with the client, must recognize this will be hard because without the hierarchy to provide the framework all the 'bad' feelings that have been projected out will come winging home.

If clinical autonomy is to be attained the principles of practice must be internalized so that they can be applied flexibly and afresh in each new situation. There will then be less need for external structures. I see clinical autonomy as incompatible with external control and with the existing system of supervision, certainly as long as it includes the policing aspect.

Can midwives carry the assertive and 'masculine' faculty of clinical autonomy with a 'feminine' empathy encouraging networking support structure to deliver the high standard of individualized, client centred care that 'Changing Childbirth' requires?

References

Association of Radical Midwives (1995). *Super-Vision: Consensus Conference Proceedings.* Hale: Books for Midwives Press.

Demilew, J. (1995). 'Examples of good supervision' in Association of Radical Midwives (Eds). *Super-Vision: Consensus Conference Proceedings.* Hale: Books for Midwives Press.

Department of Health (1993). *Changing Childbirth: The Report of the Expert Maternity Group.* London: HMSO.

Edwards, N. (1993) 'The Cumberlege Report'. *AIMS Journal.* Vol. 5, No. 3 Autumn.

Gecko (1995) 'Revitalised and healed'. *Midwifery Matters* 66, Autumn.

Halton, W. (1994). 'Some unconscious aspects of organizational life' in Obholzer, A., Zagier Roberts, V. (Eds). *The Unconscious at Work.* London: Routledge.

Hawkins, P., Shohet, R. (1989). *Supervision in The Helping Professions.* Buckingham: Open University Press

James, J. (1990). 'The role of the birth attendant'. *New Generation.* June.

Klein, M. (1975). *Envy and Gratitude.* London: Virago.

Lomas, P. (1987). *The Limits of Interpretation: What is Wrong with Psychoanalysis?* Harmondsworth: Penguin.

Menzies-Lyth, I. (1988). *Containing Anxiety in Institutions.* London: Free Association Books.

Milner, M. (1987). *The Suppressed Madness of Sane Men.* London: Tavistock Publications.

Southern, M. (1994). 'Labour and sexuality' *Midwifery Matters* 61, Summer.

Taylor, M. (1995). 'Psychodynamic counselling and therapy' in ARM (Ed). *Super-Vision: Consensus Conference Proceedings.* Hale: Books for Midwives Press.

Winnicott, D.W. (1975). *Through Paediatrics to Psychoanalysis.* London: Hogarth Press.

Index